This Old Heart of Mine:
My Inspirational Cardiac Journey

By

Chris Hillman

ISBN: 978-1-9163789-4-0

Published By: -

i2i
PUBLISHING

i2i Publishing. Manchester.
www.i2ipublishing

Dedicated to my wife Helen. Thanks for putting up with my often, bizarre behaviour, over the last two and a half years while I put this book together.

Acknowledgements

Special thanks must go to my Consultant, Mr Amal Bose who gave me my 'Second Life' and was instrumental in making the post-operative journey that enabled the writing of this book possible. For all of that, I am forever indebted to you, Sir.

Next, my sincere thanks to everyone else working at the Lancashire Cardiac Centre based at the Blackpool Victoria Hospital, for their help and enthusiasm in giving me so much of the content, time and support which has enabled me to put the book together.

I'd also like to thank all the patients who were willing to share their patient journeys with me and allowing me to include these stories in the book.

Finally, thanks must go to the British Women Pilots' Association (BWPA) and three of its members, for letting me share their career journeys.

Without you all, the book would not have been possible.

Contents

Prologue   The Lost Six hours   7

Chapter 1. The Circle of Life   13

Chapter 2. This Old Heart of Ours   33

Chapter 3. Time for a Double…Bypass   51

Chapter 4. A Return to Theatre Beckons   67

Chapter 5. What a Performance   101

Chapter 6. The Ward Round   125

Chapter 7. Second Life and a New Buddy   139

Chapter 8. Laughter in the Face of Trauma   161

Chapter 9. Female Pioneers of Change   181

Epilogue   Journey's Conclusions   205

6

Prologue

The Lost Six Hours

Thank you for picking up my book.

By reading it, you will make me one of the wealthiest people on the planet, not in monetary terms, that was never my motivation. But in the emotional wealth that comes from the feeling that you may have helped someone get through a traumatic phase in their life, or you have inspired someone to stop for a moment and question what life is really about. That's the wealth I'm talking about.

But how do you write a book? I had never written one before, my grammar is appalling, and I have no idea what phrasing means.

Then I got inspiration from Frank Sinatra and decided to do it 'My Way'.

This book is a million miles from being a literary masterpiece and it will never win any writing awards. But one thing it does have in abundance is that it's written from the heart, literally and figuratively, with a passion that I would hope is equal to any famous prize-winning author.

I hope the book will challenge your view of life and that the real stories I have included will inspire and motivate you to maximise the rest of that life. This is a book for everyone, and I do mean everyone, not just people with heart conditions.

This real-life book is written more like a novel. But unlike most novels that rely on the author's creativity to develop storylines and interesting characters, our characters are real. They are real people who have incredible stories and journeys to tell. Many have been born again, gifted a second chance in life following heart surgery.

There are amazing stories, such as a soldier who had his leg blown to pieces in 1991 during the Irish conflict. Following this, he went into an emotional meltdown and tried to commit suicide in a very bizarre way, but fortunately he failed. If that wasn't enough, he then found out he had a serious heart condition. In a very passionate interview, the soldier told me he believed he was the luckiest and happiest man on the planet!

Never before has a book been written by a patient who has been given an all-access pass to a world-class cardiac centre. This access has given me a unique insight into the dedication and professionalism of those healthcare professionals who we trust with our lives to make us healthy again.

It's not a medical book nor is it about the NHS or the cardiac department at Blackpool Victoria Hospital. It's not a book riddled with technical terms or endless statistics.

It's a book about the inspirational journey taken by those of us who have heard the words no-one ever wants to hear about the state of their heart. Seven million people in the UK and close to thirty million in the US, live with some kind of cardiovascular condition or disease every day. Probably most of the eight billion people who inhabit the planet, will know someone who has or had a heart condition.

Hopefully, it will make you laugh out loud, maybe even bring a tear to your eye but most importantly, I hope it inspires you.

I was in my sixty-seventh year and thought I was relatively fit apart from a little breathlessness. That was, until I heard the words, 'You need a double bypass and a mitral valve repair.'

On the third of January 2017 at one in the afternoon, I was put to sleep. At approximately seven-thirty in the evening, I woke up in the Cardiac Intensive Care Unit (CICU). I looked like I was wired up to a spacecraft with so many tubes, monitors, whistles and bells around me.

For the months after my surgery, emotionally, I could not overcome the incredible need to know what had happened to me during those lost six hours. I went to sleep in one physical state but woke up in a very different one. My body was not the same; I had a large scar down my chest, I had tubes coming out of my abdomen. Someone had actually been inside my body and handled the most important organ within it - incredible!

I needed to know what had happened to me.

On the incredible, life-changing journey that followed, I have interviewed consultant surgeons and reveal the personality behind the consultant mask. I have seen incredible world-class surgery being undertaken by some of the most gifted individuals on the planet. For these amazing individuals, it's just another day in the office, but for me and the patients whose lives they are saving, it's a day no words can describe.

Thanks to the amazing reception I received from the Lancashire Cardiac Centre team, I have been able to propose some rather off-the-wall experiments. For instance, we used Holter heart monitors to gain an insight into the heart performance of the surgeons themselves while performing critical procedures in theatre. The results were fascinating.

I meet the legendary American doctor Hunter 'Patch' Adams who had a Hollywood blockbuster movie made of his life, starring Robin Williams. We explore humour and laughter as a powerful medicine for coping with trauma and aiding recovery.

Most of all, I meet the patients and their families: Those people who give their complete trust to virtual strangers in the hope they can make them healthy again. The book is all about inspirational stories of the health professionals and their patients who suddenly find that heart surgery has given them a second chance, empowerment and the desire to make the most of their extended lives. I use lots of musical anecdotes and famous quotes to drive home some of the content.

Finally, I have tried to make the book interactive. At the end of each chapter, I pose a question for readers, one that hopefully you will take a few moments to consider and think about. If these questions make you come up with answers, I would love to hear about them. I ask you to send your replies to *chris@thisoldheartofmine.co.uk*

Hopefully, now that you have read these opening words, you have been inspired enough to continue to read on. I'd like to think that the book is a great read. I really hope you will too.

'Look for opportunities in every life - changing situation'

Chapter 1

The Circle of Life

'Challenges are what makes life interesting...overcoming them is what makes life meaningful'

One day in the operating theatre, I glanced at the monitors showing the patients heartbeat. I saw the beat rise and fall and thought that is exactly what life is like. We all have highs and lows in our lives, although some of us would appear to have more of one than the other. What you don't want in life is a horizontal flat line, we all know what that means!

Marcus Aurelius once said;

"We should not fear death...what we should fear is not having lived"

Mae West said;

"You only live once, however, live it right and once is enough"

Whilst I agree with her sentiment, for the most part, I do, however, believe that heart disease can give you what I'm going to call a 'Second Life'. By that, I mean a new perception on life based on the re-evaluation that can often take place after facing and dealing with a heart problem or any life-threatening illness. Many people's lives change dramatically for the better following a heart procedure. It's the sudden realisation that we are not here forever, confirmation that we will, at some stage, depart this world.

I talk much more about the concept of the

'Second Life' later.

The Hollywood actor, Antonio Banderas said, "Having a heart attack was a very positive experience, it gave me an understanding of what life is all about and what is important."

During my research for this book, I interviewed one person who emphasised this. He told me, before heart surgery, he had lived an ordinary life. By that, he meant that he had a very mundane job, drove an average car, lived in a modest house and watched a lot of television. He confessed to not having any real ambition in life.

During his post-op recovery, he was encouraged to do some walking, an activity which he began to do every day. Gradually, he introduced a bit of running to break up the monotony of walking. Feeling inspired, he then wondered about training for a marathon. As I write this, he had just returned from running the Marathon des Sables. The MDS is a six-day, 251 kilometre ultra-marathon which is the equivalent of six regular marathons in one of the world's most inhospitable locations.

He is, without doubt, a man 'born again', empowered and now living life to the full. Would he have had such a positive life-changing outcome if he had not experienced heart surgery? I very much doubt it.

This is just one example of how heart disease and life-threatening illness of any kind can have a very positive effect on the rest of your life. It can give you your self-esteem back, increase confidence, and fill you with inspiration, opening up a whole new horizon of possibilities. It feels exhilarating, breaking barriers that stood in your way before getting, albeit unwittingly, a second shot.

But what is this thing called 'life'?

Well, most of us would own up to not having thought about it in any serious way. We're all too busy running around making a living to worry about what life is really about.

A well-known quote by Ellen Goodman says:

'Normal is getting dressed in clothes that you buy for work, driving through traffic in a car that you're still paying for, in order to get to a job that you need so you can pay for the clothes, the car and the house that you leave empty all day in order to afford to live in it.'

A cynical view maybe, but I am not sure what the alternative is. Unless you're a lottery winner, one of the one percenter's, or you've made it as a movie star, a BBC Radio 2 presenter, a successful business owner, or a Premier League footballer, then Goodman's view is probably the reality.

One fact on life is set in stone. We don't need philosophers, or the population of the planet to tell us that all living creatures have two things in common: they are born, and they die. We cash in our chips, give up the ghost, check out, blink for an indefinite length of time. Whatever metaphor we use, we all know that life will come to an end. The only thing is, we don't know when.

History confirms that, as yet, no-one, no matter how rich or famous, has been able to circumnavigate life's final destination.

The first verse of Elton John's, Disney classic

song, *The Circle of Life* begins:

> *From the day we arrive on the planet,*
> *And blinking step into the sun,*
> *There's more to see than can ever be seen,*
> *More to be done than can ever be done.*

There's more to see than can ever be seen, more to be done than can ever be done. How true! What we choose to see and do whilst on the circle of life is unique to each and every one of us.

It takes a weather satellite twenty-four hours to circle the earth, set as they often are, in sun-synchronous orbit, which is to say, they pass over the same part of the earth at the same time each day, a precise and very accurate duration.

Not so precise, however, is the duration it takes for a human to complete the circle of life. I am in my seventieth year. I guess there is more of my circle completed than there is left to complete. But how much is left? I don't know. When contemplating our lives and our own personal circle, none of us truly knows.

Every day in the UK, approximately 2,000 new-borns start their journey on their circle of life and every day more than 1,600 pass on from the circle.

In the United States, those figures are a staggering 11,000 new babies with 7,500 deaths. A moving thought. Take a moment to consider.

Unfortunately, I am getting to know far too many of the 1,600 each day who depart it.

In another verse of *The Circle of Life*, the words say:

Some of us fall by the wayside,
And some us soar to the stars,
And some of us sail through our troubles,
And some have to live with the scars.

A question I have pondered on for years, is if we are, in some way, pre-programmed to be winners or losers, in good health or bad?

Of course, your lifestyle and where you live can influence your time, health and experience on the circle. In the Lion King, Simba was born to Mufasa and Sarabi, King and Queen of Pride Rock; a very privileged environment to be born into.

My journey started a little less spectacularly than Simba's. I was the proud 8lb, 11oz son of Fred and Hilda Hillman. Now, they were nothing like the King and Queen of Pride Rock and they weren't part of the elite group mentioned above.

We lived on the Ronkswood council estate in Worcester with my sister, Yvonne. We didn't have to worry whether the car tax and insurance were up to date because we never had a one to worry about. Our transport was the No. 18 or No. 28 Midland Red bus into town.

My dad was a storeman, my mum a cleaner in the local hospital. When you don't know any different, your environment becomes your world, your expectation and appreciation of life and wealth is shaped by these surroundings. It's the life you become accustomed to and accept as the norm. It's where you make your friends and acquire your life experience and skills set. It's home.

Although Worcester produced two rock stars

in Jim Capaldi and Dave Mason, both from the chart-topping rock band Traffic, it was hardly the Mecca for budding rock stars or professional footballers, both of which were my dream vocations. Unfortunately, talent and skill were required, and I was blessed with neither!

Grammar school and university were only for the top 5% in those days, which included my clever sister. For the less academically gifted, without any O-levels or GCSE's, we took on apprenticeships in the local engineering companies. That's what I did when I was sixteen.

The one thing that kept me sane during my teens was joining Worcester Canoe Club. Fortunately, we had two Olympians at the club who took me under their wing. With their coaching, I became very competitive and good enough to enter events all over Europe. I represented Britain at the 1968 World Championships at the age of eighteen.

For me, Monday to Friday was just an inconvenience on the way to the next weekend. Life was good, even if it was for just two days a week.

When you're young, life seems as though it will go on forever. Life-threatening illness, financial and relationship pressures never cross your mind. You rarely question anything, taking things as they come and expecting life to last forever. Life becomes one big adventure.

It certainly was for me. I left Worcester the day I finished my apprenticeship. I trundled down the M5 in my beaten-up green Bedford CE panel van to live the surfer lifestyle in Newquay, Cornwall.

Whilst in Newquay, I got my first taste of the entrepreneurial spirit. I needed a job that would fit in with the tides and quality of the surf. Working in a hotel with fixed hours, as most people did, would not work for me. I needed much more flexibility.

Back in the early seventies, shell lamps were extremely popular. Essentially, these were decorative wrought iron frames with seashells fitted to them. The shells had light bulbs inside to illuminate them. At the time, they were very fashionable, and everyone wanted them. In Newquay, there was a retail outlet called The Shell Shop, which sold shell lamps but were struggling to find someone to make them. A quick chat with the owner and we agreed I could come in whenever I wanted to, as long as there was enough stock available. I negotiated the fee I would get for each one I made, so the more lamps I made, the more I would earn. This was the perfect scenario for me, giving me the flexibility, I needed to work around my surfing lifestyle.

I spent two winters on the beach in Agadir, Morocco before emigrating to Australia as a '£10 Pom'. In those days, you could emigrate to Australia for just £10 providing you stayed for two years and contributed to the Australian economy. My contribution to the economy was to consume as much Penfolds wine as it was physically possible.

Later, I trained as a Samaritan's counselor and some of the life stories I heard over the phone were so traumatic and sad, it made you realise just how horrendous some people's lives are. It was also a very humbling experience to realise that, despite whatever troubles you had, your own life was a hell of a lot better than some peoples.

Many times, I took calls from distraught individuals who had just come out of a doctor's consultation having been diagnosed with a life-threatening illness. Their world had been shattered and they had to go home and deliver the devastating news to family and friends. They would phone the Samaritans to express their feelings, seeking a 3rd party companion to talk it through with, before facing family and friends. Some calls could last forty minutes, during that time I would barely say anything. My role was to listen and support them whilst they vented their feelings and came to terms with the reality of the situation.

On receiving the earth-shattering news that you have a life-threatening illness; we are prepared to hand over our bodies to complete strangers in the hope or faith that they will fix us. I remember doing exactly that with my consultant surgeon, Mr Amal Bose.

I remember the first time I met him. He had an air of confidence about him and a very calming tone to his voice. I felt relaxed in his company as he seemed to know what he was talking about. I just kept nodding as I tried to digest what he was telling me. I would suggest to anyone going into a consultation like this, take someone with you. This is so you get a second interpretation of what you are being told. The chances are your head will be spinning and you won't remember half of what is being said.

I wanted to capture inspirational stories through the lens of heart disease. I came to learn that every patient's journey is different. Where I have openly discussed my emotional trauma, other patients faced different challenges.

With permission, I was able to interview a number of them for inclusion in the book and we shall hear their stories in the following pages.

As part of my research for the book, I had the privilege to sit in on one of Mr Bose's clinics. He was seeing several patients for the first time with one pre-operative patient returning to ask more questions. The first was an eighty-three-year-old gentleman. He found it difficult to walk very far without getting out of breath. He sat down in front of Mr Bose. Mr Bose showed the man his angiogram (a type of x-ray making use of a contrast agent to visualise blood flowing through the coronary arteries and valves) and explained what surgical procedures were available.

In the forty-five minutes the gentleman spent in the room, he was never rushed, even though clinic slots for new patients are scheduled for thirty minutes. Every question was answered with precision and understanding. The gentleman, Derek, left with options to consider and no doubt a million other questions would soon come to him. His life had changed forever in those forty-five minutes. The reality of his situation had dawned.

Derek and I have become good friends as I have visited him many times since his procedure.

Later on, in a conversation I had with Mr Bose, he told me he has encountered the widest range of people in his clinics, all with a varying appreciation of why they were there. Some have no idea they have a major health issue; others want to know every little detail about what is going to happen to them.

I wanted to re-live this part of my life. The bit where you had been to your GP with a problem. They refer you to a cardiologist who would request several tests such as an angiogram and an echocardiogram. Based on the results, the cardiologist would decide as to whether you need to be considered for surgery.

I wanted to understand the apprehensions patients experience as they waited to be called in to see the consultant, so I arrived early for an appointment to interview Mr Tony Walker, one of the Consultant cardiac surgeons. I went and sat in the waiting room and observed the behaviour and body language of the patients.

In the waiting room, there were around thirty chairs all neatly positioned in groups. I counted eleven people sitting around the assembled chairs. There were five individuals and three couples waiting to be seen by the only consultant running a clinic that day.

A large flat-screen TV hung in the corner. On this particular summer day, Sue Barker was introducing the next match to be played on the Centre Court at Wimbledon, but none of the patients showed any interest, individually, they were all in their own little world.

Seeing these two very different worlds in the same room created a real dilemma. On-screen, you had Wimbledon, a world-class sporting arena where the competitors were at the peak of physical and mental fitness. To my left, I saw individuals at the other end of life's spectrum, people with real health issues.

Unlike the beaming faces in the stands at Wimbledon, the smaller crowd to my left were considerably less excited about what was about to happen.

I left for my appointment with Mr Walker.

A friend of mine is the managing director of a family business. They own four rather nice hotels in the Lake District. Simon had heart surgery three and a half years ago. He has a fascinating life story.

I arrange to meet Simon in the very luxurious new lounge of the Low Wood Bay Resort & Spa.

Patient Simon Berry - His story

Simon started by saying that it was three and a half years since his surgery under the care of Mr Andrew Duncan at Blackpool Victoria.

Simon is a devout Christian and has been so since his early twenties. Faith has been a big part of his life. I was interested to know if his faith influenced his view on his heart surgery.

He said he was aware that he was about to undertake an operation during which his whole life would be at stake, but, because of his faith and belief in an afterlife, he was completely at ease with the situation. The one thing he was concerned about, as we all are in this situation, is the people he might leave behind.

As well as his faith, the one thing Simon held dear was a strong conviction that he still had a lot to achieve. God knew that too, so he needed to survive. He saw it as a "win-win" scenario, in that, if he survived, he would have a higher quality of life to do all the things that still needed to be done. If he died, he would do so in glory and good faith and God would be waiting for him; so, he really couldn't lose.

One very cold morning, he went outside for some logs. Whilst filling the wheelbarrow, he was gripped by a severe pain down his arm. Diana, his wife was just going off for a walk with the dogs when Simon called her back and explained what had happened. As a nurse, she knew something was not right, so she took him down to the doctors for an ECG.

Reading the trace, the doctor went off to speak to someone. When he came back, he said, "Well, the good news is they don't want to rush you off in an ambulance right now. But the bad news is that first thing Monday morning, you're at Lancaster for a stress test ECG, then on Tuesday, you're at Westmorland General for an angiogram."

After the angiogram, Simon honestly thought he was going to be told he would need to take Aspirin for the rest of his life. But what he was told was, "You need bypass surgery, and soon." Stunned, Simon uttered, "Are you kidding?" Unfortunately for Simon, they weren't.

On the sixth of January 2015, Simon had his procedure. It was a success.

Since the procedure and the subsequent recovery period, Simon has gone on to achieve many of the things *he wanted to do. These include a huge multi-million-pound extension to his flagship hotel, The Low Wood Bay Resort & Spa on the shores of Lake Windermere. He has created something called 'Hi Cycling.' This is for anyone who has had a heart complication and owns an electric bike. Simon has also become the High Sheriff of Cumbria, an extremely high-profile role which demands an incredible amount of time and energy.*

It looks like Simon has been born again, twice.

If you've not been there, then it is hard to understand the emotional turmoil you go through. Amal Bose once told me despite having done thousands of heart procedures, he still has no idea what it feels like to be a patient going on the journey.

In the UK, more than 30,000 heart procedures take place each year. The success rate of elective surgery (those procedures which are planned, not emergencies) is incredibly high at more than 98%. But that doesn't stop you worrying that you might be one of the 2%, the small group that doesn't survive, as someone has to be in it!

Life, to many people, is all about exploration. Pushing the boundaries. We are an incredibly inquisitive race, never satisfied with what we have.

On the seventeenth of December 1903, life was about to change forever. Two American brothers called Orville and Wilber Wright had come up with a crazy idea. They were sure they could build a structure that was 'heavier than air' and make it travel above the ground.

They did four flights on that fateful day; the first, just twelve seconds, the last an amazing fifty-nine seconds. Look at what we have achieved in flight, not to mention space travel. All in less than a hundred and twenty years!

What the human body and spirit can tolerate always amazes me. Edmund Hilary, climbing Everest in 1953, would have had very basic clothing for coping with such severe weather conditions. He would have had none of the technology which comes as standard in today's climbing gear.

Nowadays, climbing Everest has become much easier thanks to the advancement of climbing gear and clothing.

Talking of Everest, my son Jamie and wife Jo were renewing their wedding vows at Ambleside church where they got married. For some unknown reason, I was drawn across to the church community centre where, on entry, I saw a massive pull-up banner announcing, 'Steve Watts is going to do a talk about competing in the Everest marathon…with a pacemaker!' I had to meet Steve and see if he would give me an interview.

Patient Steve Watts - His story
There is no other way of introducing Steve other than he is an ordinary man who has done extraordinary things with his life. And I do mean extraordinary.

We agree to meet at the Mortal Man, a pub in the

beautiful Troutbeck valley in the Lake District.

Over a cool larger and lime, Steve started telling me his family of six lived in a two-bedroom flat in the tough, Collyhurst part of Manchester. He makes the point that at the time, he was unaware that it was a tough estate because it was his home and the environment, he grew up in.

From a very early stage in our interview, it became clear to me that this was a guy who had talent. Not necessary a talent you could see like a footballer or an actor but a talent to see the world from a different, more creative perspective than those around him. He would definitely be moving on in life.

Move on he did. His story continues with one Saturday morning, on a solo trip into Manchester, he walked past an army recruitment office with an amazing picture of Grenadier Guards in the window. Within weeks, Steve was out of Manchester doing his induction training in Pirbright, home of the guards.

He did three tours in Northern Ireland at the peak of the troubles. On one of his trips home, he found the family to be under a considerable amount of stress, so he decided to leave the guards and return home to help manage the situation.

One day, the family got a phone call and were told to get to the hospital immediately, as his brother Bobby had died of a heart attack.

At the time, Steve never thought of having any checks on his own heart.

Steve called himself 'army fit' but read an article about a legendary Cumbrian sheep farmer called Joss Naylor. In the article, it said Joss had run one hundred miles, climbed seventy-two peaks all within twenty-four hours. In disbelief, Steve wrote to Joss and got invited to the Naylor farm in Wasdale, a remote part of West

Cumbria. Joss signed a photo for Steve before saying in a broad Cumbrian accent, "Thou need to lose sum weet. Stop smoking and get on yon fells lad."

With this instruction ringing in his ears, Steve and his wife Christina bought tracksuits and trainers. But these were no ordinary tracksuits, these were fluorescent pink. You know, the kind you find in the centre aisle of an Aldi supermarket.

An obsession had been born. But on their way to their first run, they did stop for a quick cigarette.

Steve joined Rochdale Harriers and soon became totally committed to running. He did the 'Bob Graham Round' which is sixty-eight miles over forty-two peaks with more elevation climbed than Everest.

However, that all changed. Whilst working at North Manchester General Hospital, Steve's wife Christina noticed he was pale and not looking well. She advised him to go to A&E. When he arrived, he saw the chaos there, so decided he wasn't going to stay. On his way out, he felt faint again and went back in. He remembers saying to the receptionist, "I'm not well, I think I'm here to stay." Within minutes, he was on a trolley. He thought he was dying. His thoughts suddenly reverted to his brother Bobby and what happened to him.

Steve was in the hospital for a week having many tests done. This is when he met his cardiologist and now friend, Paul Atkinson. Paul is a fellow fell runner and understanding Steve's level of fitness and training regime, said that he thought he knew what the problem was. Steve was diagnosed with Bradycardia. This is when you have a heart rate lower than sixty beats a minute and you don't get enough oxygen to your vital organs such as your brain and when that happens, you faint. Many athletes have slow heart rates, but Steve was down as low as twenty-nine and irregular.

Once again, the cardiologist, understanding the lifestyle of Steve and his fitness level, said he would set the pacemaker at forty beats a minute, in other words, if Steve's natural rhythm dipped below forty, then the pacemaker would kick in. It was agreed that forty beats a minute was enough to supply enough oxygen to all his vital organs.

From here on, Steve's life changed completely, and this is where the extraordinary achievements start to flow. As I said to him, he needs to get someone to write his autobiography because some of Steve's achievements have been nothing short of unbelievable. Through his running, he has raised in excess of £1 million for various charities.

I am always fascinated by how happy and contented people are with life, so I asked Steve if he could swap the life he has now for a multi-million-pound house on the side of Windermere, with a Bentley Continental on the driveway and all the 'boys toys,' would he? Steve smiled and said he is never happier than when he is in the hills or when he is doing his day job as a mountain guide, educating people about the Lakes, their history and discovering secret locations. I'll take that as a 'no,' you wouldn't swap then, Steve?

On the day I met Steve, my arthritis was having one of its flair ups, to the point I almost cancelled the meeting. An hour and a half in the company of this man would make anyone want to run out and climb their own Everest. Even if their Everest is pushing a trolley around a supermarket for the first time after heart surgery.

Arthritis! what arthritis.

As I mentioned above, every patient's journey is

unique. Even if you underwent the same procedure as the patient in the bed next to you, your circumstances, your physical and emotional journey will be different.

In my case, heart surgery has made me very in tune with my body. I have become highly sensitive to all the signals my body gives me. Things I might ordinarily have ignored now suddenly demand my attention and investigation.

Two years on, my emotional wellbeing has changed significantly. I feel I know what I want to achieve with the time I have left and am physically and emotionally fitter than I have ever been. I now realise that we only have one life and that it's down to us to maximise what we do with it.

In my teens, it was the era when bands were experimenting with certain illegal substances and writing enlightened songs offering an incredible insight into life. In 1973, Pink Floyd a young group of twenty-somethings wrote a song called 'Time' the words were a view on life. It was an incredible insight for guys of such a young age. Here are just a few lines from the song. It helps if you can remember the melody:

> *You are young, and life is long, and there is time to kill today*
> *And then one day you find, ten years have got behind you*
> *No-one told you when to run, you missed the starting gun*

I am fascinated by people and what they can and can't achieve in life. Thomas Edison once said he tried 10,000 times before he found the solution to the light bulb. How many of us would have given up long before then? He is also reputed to have said; he never worked a day in his life, seeing every day as an opportunity to have fun. More on 'fun' later.

Sometimes in life, we question whether as an individual we can change anything. I have never voted at a general election, my view has been, 'What difference will my vote make?'

Whilst researching the book, I started to unfold the difference one person can make on the world. I came across a fantastic quote by Apple founder Steve Jobs. It went like this:

'Here's to the crazy ones, the misfits, the rebels, the troublemakers, the round pegs in the square holes... the ones who see things differently -- they're not fond of rules... You can quote them, disagree with them, glorify or vilify them, but the only thing you can't do is ignore them because they change things... they push the human race forward, and while some may see them as the crazy ones, we see genius, because the ones who are crazy enough to think they can change the world, are often the ones who do.'

Is there such a thing as the perfect life? If there is I have yet to meet the person living it. As mentioned upfront, everyone's life and I do mean everyone's, replicates a heartbeat with high and low points. Having heart surgery can change the balance and give you many more highs than lows.

I live in the wilds of Cumbria. On a clear night, there is no light pollution other than that given out by the moon and stars. Standing beneath the Milky Way's three-hundred billion stars, I look up and ask for just one of them to send down a ray of light with the answer to what is this thing called life! I am still waiting for the answer.

Reader Question

Think about how happy and fulfilled are you with your life to date.

If you were told you had a really short time left, what would you want to achieve?

Chapter 2

This Old Heart of Ours

"You can achieve anything in life... if you put your heart and soul into it."

The heart is the most iconic organ in the body. We all have one. We all rely on one. But in reality, it's just a very unromantic, ugly pump.

Unless you have seen a real human heart, and I would hope that you haven't, then your in-built image of a heart is probably the typical symmetrical, red Valentine's shape, the one on the book cover. That's the image you should retain because the real thing is nothing like it.

The first time I saw a beating heart inside a real person was an amazing moment in my life. The surgeon had made a large incision down the middle of a patient's chest. The sternum (chest bone) was sawn open and the ribcage prized apart to expose the heart and lungs. To the theatre team, this was nothing out of the ordinary, just another day in the office. But I was rooted to the spot, overwhelmed by the realisation that this had happened to me. Here I was, no more than two feet away from a living human being, their chest wide open and the most important organ in their whole body exposed and beating before me.

To me, the heart is like a four-cylinder car engine. It has four chambers, plenty of plumbing, some valves, and a spark plug. I once mentioned this analogy to Mr Andrew Duncan, the lead consultant in the Lancashire Cardiac Centre at the

Blackpool Victoria Hospital. He fired back with, "It's nothing like a car engine. A car engine spends most of its time switched off and motionless." He continued, "The heart is about the size of your fist and can beat around 100,000 times a day. It pumps the equivalent of 2,000 gallons of blood around 60,000 miles of veins, arteries, and vessels every day and it will do that non-stop 24/7 for around 70-90 years. Nothing man-made can get close to the incredible natural ability of the heart."

Incredible though the heart certainly is, it is sadly not invincible. As I have mentioned already, I was found to have a leaky mitral valve. There are a number of valves inside the heart which allow blood to pass from one chamber to another. The valves open to allow blood to pass through and then close to prevent it flowing back where it came from. When a heart valve leaks, it is failing to close properly and so a portion of the blood flows backwards (the professionals call this 'regurgitation').

But, one condition not being enough, I also suffered from coronary artery disease. This results from the build-up of cholesterol plaque inside the arteries which supply blood to the tissues of the heart itself. This blockage obstructs the regular flow of blood to the heart muscle. This can damage the heart, which must work harder to pump blood through narrowed vessels and is a situation that can result in a heart attack.

The heart is the most iconic human organ, it's true. It is associated with love, plastered all over shop windows and gaudy cards on Valentine's Day. It also features in music and poetry, turning up in idioms and metaphors of all kinds. Here are just a few examples:

Have a heart
Heart of Glass
After my own heart
Don't go breaking my heart
My heart skipped a beat
Heart of gold
Young at heart
Close to my heart
With all my heart
Heart on his sleeve
From the bottom of my heart
A heart-stopping moment.

So many song lyrics have the word heart at their core. Mariah Carey wrote a very inspirational song called "Hero". The first verse goes like this:

There's a hero,
If you look inside your heart.
You don't have to be afraid
of what you are.
There's an answer if you reach inside your soul,
and the sorrows that you feel will melt away.

They say a picture is worth a thousand words but not if you can write words like that. Those lyrics delivered the way only Mariah Carey can, can be so moving. They can, quite literally, change your mindset forever.

I printed these words out and gave them to a man I was 'buddying' on his recovery from a heart procedure. I did it because I thought he was suffering emotionally as I did. I said to him whenever you feel a little low read these words out loud to yourself. The next time I met him he told me the words had helped him endure some dark moments of insecurity.

The heart shape is recognised the world over as a symbol of romantic love and affection, but its historical origins are difficult to pin down. Some believe the iconic image is derived from the shape of ivy leaves, which are associated with fidelity, while others contend it was modelled after breasts, buttocks, and other intimate parts of the human anatomy.

Perhaps the most realistic theory concerns silphium, a species of giant fennel that once grew on the North African coastline near the Greek colony of Cyrene. The ancient Greeks and Romans used silphium as both a food flavouring and medicine - it supposedly worked wonders as a cough syrup - but it was most famous as an early form of birth control. Ancient writers and poets hailed the plant for its contraceptive powers, and it became so popular that it was harvested into extinction by the first century A.D. (legend has it that the Roman Emperor Nero was presented with the last surviving stalk). Silphium's seedpod bore a striking resemblance to the modern Valentine's heart, leading many to speculate that the herb's associations with love and sex may have been what first helped popularise the symbol. The ancient city of Cyrene, which grew rich from the silphium trade, even put the heart shape on its money.

While the silphium theory is certainly compelling, the true origins of the heart shape may be more straightforward. Scholars have argued that the symbol has its roots in the writings of the ancient physician Galen and the still more ancient philosopher Aristotle who described the human heart as having three chambers with a small dent in the middle.

I was invited to be a guest at a talk by Professor Francis Wells, a retired but well-respected heart surgeon. He had a great admiration for the anatomical drawings of Leonardo Da Vinci. Leonardo created these illustrations in the 15th century. Try and think what it must have been like back then. No cameras, no computers, no 3D imaging. Leonardo is said to have personally dissected 30 cadavers for the sake of this groundbreaking research. Professor Wells was fascinated by the accuracy of Leonardo's drawings of the heart. During his talk, he would project a real heart and then place Leonardo's drawing alongside it for comparison. The accuracy was astonishing.

Whilst doing my research I found many alternatives as to how the shape of the Valentine's heart came about. But the above seems to be the most common. With a little bit of imagination, our actual hearts do come close to the Valentine shape. But, if you've ever seen a real human heart, it's just as unattractive as any other organ inside you. Veiny, ugly, and gnarled. Even cleaned up it's raw, visceral, and thoroughly unromantic.

Heart disease is the number one killer of men and women in Britain today, closely followed by cancer. Heart disease kills one in four of us. That equates to 170,000 deaths a year or one death every three minutes. Every one of us will know someone who has heart disease or a heart condition like atrial fibrillation. Recent statistics issued by the British Heart Foundation (www.bhf.org.uk) highlight the following staggering facts which were correct at the time of writing.

On a daily basis in the UK:

- 460 people will lose their lives to some form of cardiovascular disease (CVD).
- 115 of these people will be younger than 75.
- 7 million people live a daily battle with CVD.
- 250+ people will be admitted to a hospital as the result of a heart attack.
- 180 people will die from a heart attack.
- 12 babies will be diagnosed with a heart defect.

The British Heart Foundation is the biggest UK charity for anything to do with heart conditions and disease. The BHF should be the first stop for anyone wanting further information and support on heart welfare. Their vision is:

'A world free from the fear of heart and circulatory diseases. A world without heartbreak.'

Here are some incredible facts about the BHF, an organization founded in 1961, summarized from their website.

The BHF aims to ensure that at least 70p of every £1 raised will be available to spend on life-saving work, and the balance is invested to grow their income. This year 72p in every £1 raised was available to spend on charitable activities; the remaining 28p was invested to generate our income.

Research - Last year, they awarded an incredible £128.2m in life-saving medical research grants that will improve how we prevent, diagnose and treat heart and circulatory diseases. They've committed to funding a billion pounds of ground-breaking research over the next ten years to deliver significant breakthroughs that will help save and improve the lives of millions of people across the UK and globally.

Fundraising - Their generous supporters helped them to raise an incredible £138.1m towards their life-saving work. This includes £84.9m left to the BHF in legacies, and £53.2m raised by generous supporters through community fundraising activities, corporate partnerships, events, major gifts and mass participation events.

Retail - Their 732 BHF shops across the UK generated £22.9 million in profit by collecting, sorting and selling around 74,000 tons of goods over the last year. While the shops and stores remain vibrant community hubs, the BHF's growing online activity saw 143,000 items sold on eBay, helping to bring in £5.4m across eBay and online sales.

Heart Support Groups - Nearly 300 affiliated Heart Support Groups bring hope and a healthier lifestyle to thousands of patients and carers across England and Wales.

These groups are open to anyone with any kind of heart condition as well as their partners and families.

In the 1960s, it was more like 70% of people who had a heart attack would die. Today, the numbers have reversed, so that 70% now survive from a heart attack if they get treatment in time. However, seven hundred young, fit individuals still die each year due to cardiac arrest. When post-mortems have been carried out there would appear to be no anatomical problems within the heart.

A famous case was that of Premier League footballer Fabrice Muamba. His book I'm Still Standing recalls the events of the seventeenth of March 2012. It was the FA Cup semi-final at White Hart Lane, home to Tottenham Hotspur. Fabrice was a Bolton Wanderers player but had been struggling to keep a regular place in the team. Yet on this day, his manager, Owen Coyle, had put his faith in Fabrice. He was in the starting team.

This was a massive day, not just for Fab, but for the entire club as things had not been going well throughout that season. This was an opportunity for the club to make some serious cash as well as give their loyal fans something to cheer about. The game starts and it's soon 1-1.

Twenty-five minutes into the game and Fab gets a tingly headache. It only lasts a couple of minutes. Several minutes pass by and Fab is reading the game. Suddenly, a much stronger headache returns. It feels like the right side of his skull is being crushed. The game is moving and Fab needs to get back to defend but his legs tell him they can't move. Seconds later, Fab hits the turf headfirst, totally out of control. Doctors dash onto the pitch without the approval of the referee. It's plain to all watching that Fab is in a bad way.

Fab had suffered a massive cardiac arrest. For the next seventy-eight minutes, Fab was all but dead as they tried and tried through CPR and defibrillation to get his heart beating again. Sitting in the crowd was Dr Andrew Deaner, a consultant cardiologist at King George Hospital and the London Chest Hospital. Recognising what was happening, he quickly made his way onto the pitch and arranged for Fab to be taken to a specialist hospital. After seventy-eight minutes of resuscitation attempts, his heart miraculously started again.

Fab's heart was found to have no physical defects but the trauma it had sustained meant his playing days were over.

During the time I was writing this book another very famous footballer died of a heart attack. Ray Wilkins, formerly of Chelsea, Manchester United, and England had a heart attack at home. He was rushed to hospital but sadly died. Ray was an incredibly nice guy. I know because I had the pleasure of working with him in 1980. Some footballers let themselves go when they stop playing but Ray stayed in football as a manager and as a coach and kept himself fit. It's a terrible mystery why so many fit sportsmen and women suffer in this manner, having experienced no problems before the tragic event. I interview a young triathlete in a later chapter to try and understand this phenomenon.

There are various causes of heart disease and some people seem to experience this disease more than others.

Many years ago, I was able to spend a whole month living with a nomadic Masai tribe in the Kenyan bush. Now their lives and material assets are completely different from the lifestyles of the rich and famous, and probably everyone reading this book. Heart disease is virtually unknown within Marsai tribes.

The Masai live in what they call Manyattas. A Manyatta is a group of mud huts surrounded by a twig fence to stop wild animals getting in and stealing the sheep and goats. Wealth in Masai terms is all about the number of sheep and goats a family owns.

In the late sixties and early seventies, Jomo Kenyatta, the President of Kenya, tried to get the nomadic Masai to stay in one place and build Shamba's (a Shamba is a smallholding or farmstead). He even supplied Land Rovers for them to use.

One day on a walkabout, the Masai took me to the remains of a Land Rover. They told me they would drive them until they ran out of petrol. When that happened, they went back to what they do best: walking. Cardiac disease within the Masai is very rare, maybe we should learn from their lifestyle.

On the face of it, the Masai have very little by way of material wealth, they might even be considered primitive by some standards.

I spent many a day sat under an Acacia tree laughing and joking with them whilst their sheep and goats grazed. As long as the sheep and goats were safe and their families were malaria free, then they were incredibly content with life. They are some of the happiest and most contented people I have ever met.

On arriving home from Kenya, I could barely get through the front door. The gas bill, car tax, TV license, and several other bills had piled up blocking my entrance. I stood and wondered... who had the life question figured out, me or the Masai? Jambo!! ('Hello' in Swahili).

My own involvement with cardiovascular disease began at home. One night we were relaxing in the cottage when my wife, Helen said she didn't feel well. As she was sat on the sofa, she told me her vision was getting 'weird'. She looked scared and begged me not to leave her.

As Helen is as fit as the proverbial butcher's dog, I knew this was something serious. I called an ambulance immediately. The first person to appear was a 'first responder'. When you live way out in the country like we do you must rely on people in the community who have completed a first responder course while waiting for the paramedics to arrive.

Our nearest A&E department is some thirty-five miles away in Lancaster. Once we arrive, we are shown straight in. By this time the symptoms have passed but Helen is still emotionally unsettled. The young registrar looking after Helen arranged many tests, all to identify the cause of this episode which had left us both shaken.

Several hours later, Helen was given the all-clear, but the doctor had set up more tests for the following week. She suspected Helen had experienced a Transient Ischaemic Attack or TIA. TIA's are often described as a 'mini-stroke' producing similar symptoms to a stroke but usually lasting only a few minutes and typically causing no permanent damage. TIA's are taken very seriously as they can be the harbinger of a more severe incident to follow.

Now, let's assume you get admitted to hospital and are found to require the services of a surgeon. What does a surgeon do? Well, a cardiothoracic surgeon is someone who specialises in surgical procedures inside the thorax, which is the chest cavity that houses the heart and lungs. Within cardiothoracic surgery, there are specific domains of expertise. In fact, the term "cardiothoracic" is a compound expression referring to both cardiac and thoracic specialisms. Cardiac surgery specifically addresses problems relating to the heart while thoracic surgery addresses problems relating to the rest of the chest cavity, typically the lungs and oesophagus. Some surgeons perform both cardiac and thoracic procedures. Others specialise in one or the other.

At Blackpool, cardiothoracic surgeons tend to be in theatre two to four days a week, performing roughly two or three procedures a day. Cardiothoracic surgeons bear witness to the immediate and often life-changing results of their work. When asked why they chose to work in a cardiac environment, many said it gave them a tremendous sense of personal satisfaction to see very poorly people given back to living their lives.

The speciality is relatively young, historically speaking. But since the end of the Second World War, cardiothoracic surgery has seen accelerated growth alongside rapid technological developments. Indeed, there are now even robots that can assist with cardiac surgical procedures.

During my visits to Blackpool, I have met several remarkable trainees at various stages on their career path, many of whom we will meet throughout the course of this book.

Blackpool is a teaching hospital, helping aspiring professionals to hone their skills. The cardiac centre itself, runs a number of programmes in collaboration with nearby universities.

One of these programmes at the Blackpool Victoria Hospital is organised by Mr Antony Walker which gives medical students at the beginning of their career the opportunity to experience cardiac surgery first-hand.

Consultant Cardiac Surgeon Mr Walker – His story

Tony Walker is a highly qualified and respected consultant cardiothoracic surgeon based at Blackpool Victoria Hospital.

Apparently, he does not believe that you can do both cardiac and thoracic surgery, although some of his colleagues would disagree. He uses the expression "jack of all trades, master of none." So, he decided to become a master of cardiac surgery.

He's been a consultant at Blackpool since 2012. Before that, he was at the Leeds General Infirmary (or "LGI" as it is known).

Mr Walker has done considerable research in heart and lung transplants, genetics, immunology, growing smooth muscle cells from bits of the vein (this is a man who kept telling me he was not clever and anyone could be taught to do what he does!) Although the research wasn't what he initially wanted to do, he ended up loving it. He uses the knowledge and skills he gained from that period to make his work as a mentor more challenging and interesting.

To get a surgeon's job, he needed a training position. To get that, he needed to have gone beyond the basics, obtaining a higher degree. He acquired both.

One of Tony's strengths is that he is always probing, asking himself and his colleagues, "Why do it this way?" He is always in pursuit of a better way of working, something he impresses on the trainees he is responsible for. He says it's hard to have integrity and honesty if you don't question yourself and your processes daily. His intention is to deliver the best service possible.

Unlike other surgeons, I have interviewed, Mr Walker never had a eureka or light bulb moment about becoming a cardiac surgeon. His dad, however, did have two heart attacks over a couple of years which may have sown an unconscious seed or two.

He recalls reading Stephen Covey's, "The 7 Habits of Highly Effective People." One of those is to "start with the end in mind." For Mr Walker, the end was to be a cardiac surgeon. All that was needed was to fill in the gaps.

Much to his wife Jenny's annoyance, money has never been a big motivator, although surgeons do earn considerably more than most of us. In the corporate world, the same sacrifice, dedication, and skill level would deliver a much greater financial return but would not offer the incredible emotional satisfaction of saving someone's life. That feeling must be priceless!

One question I have asked everyone I have interviewed is, "What is the meaning of life?" The responses have been fascinating.

When I asked Mr Walker this question, he mentioned Dr Lockhart's response when I had sprung it on him mid-procedure. Dr Lockhart is an anaesthetist with more than thirty-one years' experience at Blackpool Victoria. He said the meaning of life was, "To do what's right." This is an interesting answer, and an appropriate one considering he was in theatre at the time and totally focused on the patient he was responsible for.

This response had struck a chord with Tony as, having work in one location and family in another, it's hard to do what's right for everyone.

After a few seconds thought, he came up with the reason why he had dedicated his life to this work, making the many sacrifices you have to make to become a top cardiac surgeon. He said it is to help people make the most of their lives and be able to improve the quality of what they can do. If the people I have interviewed weren't so honest, passionate and professional, I would think this was a well-rehearsed answer as several interviewees have responded similarly.

Although Mr Walker didn't come up with a slick one-sentence answer to the question, I do feel he would have given it considerable thought when he went back to his temporary Blackpool residence that night.

To finish my interviews, I try and bring things back to more light-hearted themes. Although for me, the answers can often be quite revealing and give you a unique insight into the personality of the interviewee.

The question I always ask is, "What is your favorite song or piece of music?" He responded that it depends on the mood he is in. Yesterday in the theatre it was 'the greatest football anthems ever.' Understandable, I suppose, as we were right in the middle of the World Cup. When he got home that night, it was Mozart's Requiem, because it reminded him of his choirboy days.

I also ask, "What is your favorite team?" This reply was much snappier, "Theatre 2 on a Monday morning."

Great answer, Tony.

Alma, someone we shall meet and find more about later in the book, had been waiting patiently outside to see Mr Walker. She wanted to let him know she had proposed him for an award for outstanding service.

At this point, I depart and leave Mr Walker with his adoring fan.

Have you ever bought a new car and suddenly noticed how many of the same there are? In the same way, following my surgery, I found the heart everywhere. In shop windows. On the radio. On the internet.

I was driving up the M6 the other day passing Tebay, a small village just a dozen miles away from where I live. I have driven this section of the M6 hundreds of times. But on this day, and I can't fathom out why, but my attention was drawn to the left side of the carriageway. What I saw hit me like a brick wall (and almost the car behind me too, as I braked hard). In a field, just a couple of hundred metres away was a massive heart-shaped wood. How could I have not seen this in the forty years I have lived in Cumbria? Apparently, it dates back to the early 1800s. Some stories of the wood say it was planted as a memorial to a young soldier. Another says it was planted by a farmer who wanted to show his love for his wife. The current landowner says it's just a wood which, owing to the walls it is planted around, looks like a heart. Whatever the truth it still strikes you like a heart when you drive past.

No matter who you are, a rock star, a Premier League footballer, a checkout assistant in a supermarket, or a first-time author like me, we all have one thing in common: we all need our hearts to keep beating.

I was watching a programme on TV the other day about cosmetic surgery and the incredible amounts of money people are prepared to pay to create their ideal exterior image. Some had spent years planning their procedures, travelling the world in search of surgeons who could create the image they craved.

As I watched, I remembered something Mr Andrew Duncan said to me, "Nothing man-made can compare to the beauty of a healthy human heart." You can see why I call him the Grand Master.

Reader Question

Buy a heart monitor and twice a day over a one-week period, write down your heart rate and blood pressure numbers.

Are these important performance measurements normal?

Chapter 3

Time for a Double...Bypass

*The trauma of the journey will never
compare to the empowerment of recovery*

There was a great song in the eighties by *The
Human League* called 'Human.' The first verse went
like this:

> *I'm only human,*
> *Of flesh and blood, I'm made.*
> *Human, born to make mistakes.*

Born to make mistakes is exactly what I
thought of the consultant who told me I needed a
double bypass and a mitral valve repair. As far as I
was concerned, I was fit I didn't need heart surgery.
I was just a little out of breath, that's all.

My cardiac journey began on a beautiful
afternoon in July 2012. The wind was low, and the
sun was warming our backs. Helen and I were out
on a bike ride when we came to a hill. Hills are
something you can't avoid if you live in Cumbria.
As we started the climb, I noticed Helen was
disappearing away up the hill while I seemed to be
puffing like a racehorse. Though Helen is
extremely fit I am normally able to keep up with
her. Something wasn't right!

We got back home, and I promptly forgot
about it.

A couple of days later, I had an appointment
with a rheumatologist. She did some routine tests

and happened to take my pulse. The doctor looked puzzled. So, she took it again, and again. I could see she was becoming concerned, so I asked what the problem was. My pulse was very erratic, she told me, before suggesting I have an ECG. "A what?" I replied. "An ECG will print out a trace to see how your heart is performing," she said. I was sent for one that afternoon.

Now an ECG involves putting electrodes mostly around your chest and a couple on your ankles. I swear they only put the ones on your ankles to see if you have clean socks on. You are asked to lie still while the machine does its thing (technical term), then suddenly, it starts chuntering away and printed out a long sheet with lots of graphs on it. One of them shows the rhythm of your heart. Ideally, your heart should be in what is called sinus rhythm, beating at regular intervals between 60-100 beats per minute. If your heart is beating irregularly this is called an arrhythmia, of which there are many kinds. I was found to be in atrial fibrillation (AF) where the upper chambers of my heart were beating quickly and irregularly, out of sync with the rest of the heart.

A week later, I was seeing a cardiologist at my local hospital. He reviewed my ECG results and suggested I needed a cardioversion. Again, not being the brightest human on the planet my immediate response was, "a cardio what?" He explained that a cardioversion aims to get your heart back into a regular rhythm by giving it an electrical shock. So how do you shock the heart, I asked? "Have you ever watched *Casualty* on telly?" He said. "You know when someone dies, and they try to resuscitate them by putting two pads on their chest and then shocking them? Well, that's similar to a cardioversion." The sympathetic doctor had noticed my stirring anxiety. "Don't worry you won't be awake when we do it." We put you to sleep for just a few minutes while it's done."

I return home in disbelief and wait for the letter of appointment to drop through the door. It was two months later when it arrived, the date confirmed. When the day came, Helen dropped me off and I went up to the cardiac ward. Cardioversions only take place on certain days in the month in my local hospital. From the number of people in the waiting room, I concluded it was an in-demand procedure.

As people disappeared, my apprehension grew. It seemed that the person giving the 'zap' was not a doctor but a trained nurse.

"Chris Hillman", a nurse shouted out. The time had come. I barely had time to quiz the nurse when we had arrived at our destination, the anaesthetic room.

I walked in and jumped on the bed. Dave, the specialist nurse practitioner, talked me through what was going to happen. The next thing I remember was waking up. I looked at the clock. It had barely been fifteen minutes since I had left the waiting room. "All done," said a nurse. You're back in rhythm.

You have to stay on the ward for a few hours afterwards for observations and to recover from your brief anaesthetic. As part of your recovery, they offer you a cup of tea and a slice of toast. I don't think I have ever had a cup of tea or a slice of toast that has tasted that good.

For two years, my heart behaved itself. I was back to keeping up with Helen on the hills. *Life was good!* And then, suddenly, all the previous symptoms returned: shortness of breath, falling asleep in the chair, a feeling like I had no vitality at all.

Another trip to the cardiologist confirmed I was back in AF and second cardioversion was booked. Again, it was successful and the tea and toast just as delicious as the first time.

Unfortunately, I stayed in sinus rhythm for less than a year. By this time, I was finding the whole situation very frustrating. I desperately wanted to get to the bottom of it and to get it sorted once and for all. I felt oppressed, living under this morbid shadow, and sorely wished I could get back to doing the things I had always done and wanted to do.

Several months later, I found myself over at the Lancashire Cardiac Centre in Blackpool for an angiogram. Although I didn't know this beforehand, an angiogram is a type of x-ray used to obtain images of your coronary arteries. They utilise a contrast dye to highlight the flow of blood and reveal abnormalities within the arteries and valves. At the conclusion of the test, I was asked if I had ever had any chest pains to which I replied "No." "That's surprising", I was told, "As you have significant narrowing of two of your main vessels." I was also to learn that I had a leaking mitral valve. The news hit me like a double-decker bus.

Generally, cardiac patients start by going to their GP who would ordinarily refer you on to a cardiologist. Cardiologists are medical experts who specialise in the study and care of the heart. A cardiologist is not a surgeon, but some will perform minimally invasive procedures such as a transvenous pacemaker implantation, more commonly referred to as a TAVI. When a condition warrants surgical intervention, the cardiologist will then refer you on to a cardiac surgeon. And so, in April 2016, I had my first consultation with Mr Bose, a consultant cardiac surgeon responsible for the Cumbria area.

During this consultation he outlined what needed doing. But at that moment in time, my condition was not life-threatening.

Some time had passed. It was now the second of January 2017 and I was at home celebrating my birthday. At four-thirty, the phone rang and turned my world upside down. It was Phyllis, Mr Amal Bose's secretary, asking if I could come into the hospital in the morning. "Of course," I replied, "But what for?" The response followed: "Your procedure!"

Now, this came as a shock for many reasons: First of all, it was January and the NHS was undergoing its winter bed crisis. Secondly, this was less than fourteen hours before I was due to go into theatre!

This situation, I must stress, is not the norm. Elective surgery patients ordinarily get several weeks' notice and have a pre-op medical a week or so before their procedure. However, things happen. Sometimes, patients get sick and are unable to proceed. Sometimes patients pull out at the last minute. Whatever the reason there is still a surgeon and a whole team who must operate. The show must go on.

My life was suddenly in turmoil. I hadn't seen our three kids or spoken to them. Helen and I had not spoken about the future and what might be. So many questions, so little time to answer them. That night I didn't sleep for worrying.

It's six o'clock in the morning and we are in the car heading for Blackpool. It's a quiet hour and fifteen minutes' drive. With Helen beside me, we are in our own little worlds. We arrive with barely a word spoken. To get to the main entrance from the multi-story car park, it's just a short walk across a pedestrian walkway. We pass through a large rotating door and arrive in the foyer with its huge vaulted ceiling. It is a hive of activity.

To the left, as you enter is a row of retail outlets including Costa Coffee, WH Smith's, and Marks and Spencer. To the right is Lloyd's pharmacy. At the centre is a glass lift, the type you see in very classy hotels, flanked by escalators and a staircase leading to a mezzanine. The floor is polished white stone which must take hours of upkeep to keep it in such pristine condition. Standing in the middle of the space is a group of volunteers wearing tangerine polo shirts, the same colour as Blackpool F.C, the local club, made famous by the late, great Stanley Matthews. I gather they're meant to stand out so that they can be identified by lost and bewildered souls like Helen and me.

We approach one of them and say we're looking for the Lancashire Cardiac Centre in Area 12. Now Area 12 is a little bit of a walk away. A very courteous lady volunteer gave us directions which sounded like a route march.

We make our way through the winding corridors and up one floor to Same-Day Admissions, just opposite Ward 38. On arrival, we are greeted by a courteous nurse called Dawn who tells me she needs to carry out some tests before I shower and put the glamorous NHS gown on.

The anaesthetist came in and introduced himself as Mike. Mike is the guy who's responsible for keeping me alive whilst Mr Bose is working his magic on my heart. Mike asks a lot of questions to get a feeling of my general health and what might be needed during the procedure.

I then sit with Helen in a small waiting room with several other patients. The time is around nine o'clock and I am advised that I am second on the list. So, depending on how the first procedure goes, I could be waiting into the afternoon. I now find myself saddled with plenty of time to think. The silence is broken on the rare occasion with idle chat but for the main, we are all contemplating what the next few hours have in store for us.

At midday, nurse Dawn came through to inform me that the moment had arrived. The weight of it all came crashing down. Trembling, I make a teary goodbye to Helen before sitting down in a wheelchair to be taken up to the theatre.

My wheelchair driver took a right turn and then a left and suddenly we are in the corridor. My senses alive, I realise how cold it is. We turn left and travel just a few yards before we come to the big stainless-steel lift. We enter and my driver pushes the button to take us up to the second floor. A few seconds later, the lift shunts to a halt and the big shiny doors slide open. I am completely overwhelmed! I am almost oblivious to my surroundings. Are these the last few moments of my life, I wonder? My anxiety is interrupted by the command to enter the anaesthetic room.

The room is tiny. It has a bed and enough room to walk around but that's about it. Mike, the anaesthetist is there and he asks me to jump up onto the bed. The back is up for now, so I am sitting up facing the wall. Mike tries to explain what he is doing but my mind is already saturated. I am in another world.

The last thing I remember is saying to Mike "Please make sure I see your ugly face in a few hours." This was probably not the wisest thing to say to the person who is responsible for keeping you alive, especially as Mike is far from ugly! But I cannot emphasise enough how abnormal, how volatile, my emotional state was at this point. It makes you react in unpredictable ways and the staff, fortunately, are very sensitive to this. Suddenly, my eyes felt heavy. The lights went out.

Mr Amal Bose, my surgeon, the man who was about to give me a new life, my 'Second Life', had an interesting start to his own life and career.

Consultant Cardiac Surgeon Mr Bose - His story
The son of Indian parents who came to Britain in the sixties, Amal Bose's mum was a doctor and his dad worked in finance and accountancy. They came to Britain because his mum wanted to do a post-graduate medical qualification. The plan was to stay for just a couple of years. They never went back to India.

Amal was born in London but grew up in Llanelli in west Wales until 1988, when he went back to London to attend St George's Hospital medical school.

Young Amal's introduction to the world of medicine began when his mum organised work experience for him with a surgeon. Back then, work experience was a lot easier to organise, none of the stifling Health and Safety nonsense we have to deal with today. Students had more access and were allowed to do so much more than their counterparts do today.

Inspired by this experience, he realised that surgery was what he wanted to do. His mum told him he would never be rich as a surgeon, but he would always be in demand and be able to enjoy a comfortable middle-class standard of living.

After six years at medical school, he decided he needed to travel, so applied for a job in Australia. He ended up in Queensland and spent two years in Brisbane completing his general surgical training.

It was in Australia where he got his first post in cardiothoracic surgery. He was drawn to cardiothoracic surgery because it demanded a high degree of skill and intensive care. He also made the point that there were no unpalatable elements such as bowels or gangrene.

Cardiac surgery is very meticulous and involves taking care of highly dependent patients as well as treating patients in critical need of lifesaving surgery.

When he came back to the UK, he secured a junior post at Blackpool Victoria Hospital but openly admits he didn't have a clue where Blackpool was and had to look it up on a map (no Google back then). He worked for a year in Blackpool before departing for Harefield for two and a half years.

He did a higher degree at University College, London where he spent two years immersed in research, killing rats. He spent many an hour in the coffee room contemplating why his experiments weren't working. However, something very positive came out of this time, as it was over one of these cups of coffee that he met his partner.

After two years of completing his research, it took another two years to write it up. At this point, Mr Bose had reached the grand old age of thirty-four.

After a brief eight-week stint in Swansea, Amal got a locum post in Newcastle. By now it was 2004. In 2006 they gave him a full training post. In 2010, he went to Sydney to St. Vincent's Hospital to study heart transplants. In 2011, he came back to Britain to finish his exams and look for a job in transplants. It was during this period that he was approached by former colleagues at Blackpool Victoria to take on a temporary locum role which turned into becoming a consultant.

Before undertaking this journey, I would expect the public perception of what an anaesthetist does to be similar to mine. I thought all they did was give you an injection to put you to sleep and that was it, job done. How wrong could I be? Anaesthetists are extremely clever people. Their knowledge of anatomy and physiology is nothing short of staggering. Where the surgeon is a 'master of repairing' the heart, the anaesthetist is the oracle for everything else.

Their contact with the patient will start at the pre-operative assessment. This takes place in the hospital about a week to a fortnight before the procedure. A number of investigations are carried out including a range of blood tests, swabs, and a chest x-ray. The anaesthetist will want to know many pieces of information including how much you weigh, if you smoke or drink and what medications you take. This is to help them determine how you will take to anaesthesia and whether there are likely to be any complications either in theatre or during your recovery.

On the morning of your admission, it's the anaesthetist you will most likely see before your procedure. They need to check your circumstances have not changed and may recap on the procedure you are about to undertake to make sure you understand the situation. The next time you see them will be in the anaesthetic room.

During the procedure, as the surgeon concentrates on fixing the heart, the anaesthetist is responsible for monitoring all our vital signs. On screens all around the theatre, you can see readouts of the patient's heart rate, blood pressure etc etc. The heart itself is visualised by means of a transoesophageal echocardiogram probe (TOE) for which the anaesthetist is also responsible. Cardiac procedures can take a long time, sometimes much longer than anticipated, so the anaesthetist has to maintain an open dialogue with the surgeon to keep the patient sedated should the procedure last longer than expected.

Once the patient is transferred from theatre to the CICU, they become the responsibility of the anaesthetist on the ward and the numerous dedicated professionals that work on the ward across the shift pattern. An anaesthetist is always scheduled to work on intensive care to check on the patients.

I have zero recollection of the six hours I was anaesthetised, my lost six hours. I cannot even recall dreaming during that time. I asked other patients whether they could remember dreaming and none of them could.

Some patients gain consciousness very quickly after surgery and find themselves awake even before entering the intensive care ward. I am told that older patients take a bit longer to regain consciousness. I was one of those.

Waking up after major surgery can be a very strange experience. Initially, you have no idea what has happened. The first thing I recall is a feeling of rising out of dense fog. As the seconds passed, I started to see shapes moving around me, but I could not make out what they were. A few more moments and my hearing also returned. Suddenly, I was in a world of sound I wasn't aware I'd slipped out of. But what were these sounds? I could not understand anything I was hearing.

I was fighting to grasp this strange environment. More time passed and the fog became a little less dense. From my grogginess, I could now make out outlines of nurses, machines and a number of tubes attached to my body. I wondered, "Where am I?" I was still unable to appreciate exactly what had happened to me.

A few seconds more and I experienced an incredible flash of realisation: I'd made it! I was alive! I could not begin to express how this felt, though I am sure anyone who has experienced it knows exactly what I am talking about.

Drifting in and out of consciousness is the norm for the first few hours in the Cardiac Intensive Care Unit (CICU) as the anaesthetic drugs wear off. Every time you gain consciousness, you find yourself with greater awareness of your surroundings and your situation.

Your own personal nurse will enter into conversation with you to assess how you are and where you might have pain. They are an incredibly dedicated group of health professionals who over a three-shift period are there to take care of you on a 1:1 ratio 24/7.

Fortunately, I spent the minimum amount of time on CICU and was soon ready to move down to the ward. This was good news for all concerned as it meant my recovery was going to plan and also the CICU bed I had occupied could be made available for the next patient. I was moving to Ward 38, the cardiac surgical ward I had passed on my way in when this incredible odyssey had begun.

Ward 38 looked like a more conventional ward than the one I'd just come from. That said, the impeccable personal care continued. Physiotherapists soon arrived to start my recovery, returning my mobility stage by stage. They wanted to get me moving as soon as possible and before I knew it, I was pacing, with supervision, up and down a nearby flight of stairs. I remember one day I felt good enough to take a walk away from the ward by myself. When Mr Bose came to do his ward round, he found me missing!

Four days later, I was deemed ready for home and so Helen came to collect me. I was so looking forward to being in my own home with the surroundings I knew. That said, it was like leaving the hospital with your firstborn. For a few days post-surgery, you have the security of a hospital and top-quality healthcare professionals available to you. Now you are about to take that leap into the unknown, fending for yourself. But I still couldn't wait to get back to a place I knew.

The next few weeks went by and, step by step, my fitness and mobility was returning with each passing day.

But however well the physical recovery was going, I was starting to experience emotional turmoil. Questions like, "What had happened to me? What trauma had my body gone through?" Someone, namely Amal Bose and his team, had been inside my body and had tinkered with my heart. I couldn't stop thinking about what had happened to me in those lost six hours between one-thirty and seven-thirty on the third of January 2017.

As the weeks went by, the need to know became almost obsessive. Unless you have been through a similar thing this may seem like a strange and trivial thing to be obsessive about. I looked everywhere for information. I googled it, looked on websites, got some valuable information off the British Heart Foundation website. Yet, ideally, I wanted to talk to someone, another patient who had experienced what I had experienced. I wanted to ask them if the way I was feeling was normal.

After a couple of months, I got to the point where I realised the need to know what had happened to me would literally drive me insane. I felt compelled to contact Mr Bose and arrange a meeting to discuss my dilemma and what I hoped we could do about it. On the drive down, I started to worry about what I was going to propose. Would the reasons behind it seem a little bizarre, even trivial? After all, people were having heart procedures every day and getting on with life. But were they?

I met Mr Bose in his office, a short distance from the theatre where it all happened. He greeted me with a smile and a handshake and invited me to sit down. As I did, I embarrassed myself by cracking my head against his bookcase. Amal, a true master of wit, said I should be more careful, or I'd end up getting admitted again. His humour put me at ease.

I explained my situation and tried my best to express the emotional turmoil I had been suffering with. I told him how I couldn't deal with not knowing what had happened to me during those six hours.

As my story unfolded, I became somewhat emotional. I glanced over at Mr Bose who was listening intently. He sympathised with my situation and showed great sensitivity. I asked about the possibility of being able to relive what had happened to me by seeing someone else go through a similar surgical procedure. I also expressed my disappointment that I could not find any place which could offer me the post-operative emotional support I needed.

Mr Bose offered to speak with senior management to see if we could get permission for me to observe a similar procedure to mine.

Eight weeks later, with all security checks completed, I was finally granted permission to observe a procedure. I proposed to write about my experiences as a means of coming to terms with what had happened to me. The idea snowballed. Before I knew it and not having written anything of such magnitude, I had started to write a book about my journey and those of other patients and healthcare professionals.

Reader Question

Think about the most traumatic experience you have had in your life so far.

What lessons did you learn from it?

Chapter 4

A Return to Theatre Beckons

'Life is the biggest theatre there is'

"A horse, a horse, my kingdom for a horse!" Probably one of Shakespeare's most famous lines from one of his most famous plays, Richard III. A line heard in many theatres, but perhaps out of place in the theatre I was heading to.

Today is a big day for me. I am going to observe Mr Bose performing two open-heart procedures.

I woke up at five o'clock in the morning feeling a mixture of emotions, excited by what I was about to experience but also worried that I might make a complete fool of myself and keel over at the first sight of blood. I get dressed, have a hearty breakfast as advised, and drink lots of water to help stop me from fainting.

Taking a lungful of the sharp Cumbrian morning air, I climb in the car and head off down the bumpy track that leads to and from our humble little cottage in the wilds of Selside, Cumbria.

The journey to the hospital is about an hour and a quarter so I left myself two hours to arrive by eight o'clock, the time I was asked to arrive. I drive my wife Helen crazy as I always leave way ahead of what most people would see as an acceptable time. I am paranoid about being late.

On the way, I listen to Chris Evans on the Radio. I like Chris Evans because he's a thinker. Today, he is exploring time and the claim that there can't be any past or any future. The future is always that which has not yet taken place and the past has already gone. Therefore, there can only be the present.

Thinking about this dilemma helped the journey pass quite quickly and I am soon parking up in the hospital's multi-storey car park. As I head across to the main entrance of the hospital, I start to focus on the day ahead. My chaperone for the day is to be Dr Dale Watson. Dr Watson is head of cardiac anaesthesia at the hospital and I am to be under his supervision. As I arrive at the agreed location. Dr Watson also appears, in Lycra cycle gear! Now most men I know should never go anywhere near Lycra but clearly Dr Watson keeps himself in shape and is one of the very few men who can do Lycra justice.

I do as I am told and follow him into the changing room. He grabs a set of green trousers and a top, commonly known as scrubs, along with a headwear and a pair of clogs. He tells me to take everything off except my underpants and socks and to change into this clinical attire. While I do this, Dr Watson disappears off to the shower, a daily ritual after his cycle ride in from Lytham, St. Annes.

I put the green scrubs on and, suitably dressed, I look like a real health professional. I feel enormously empowered. But I soon come down to Earth as I find myself struggling to tie the headwear at the back of my head.

I follow Dr Watson into the coffee room. It looks very similar to an ordinary staff room except everybody is similarly dressed in scrubs. There is a kitchen to the left and a vending machine in the far corner. It is very busy at this time in the morning.

I am introduced to a lady called Gill, or Registrar Ms Gill Hardman, to give her professional title. Dale tells me she is a trainee surgeon under the guidance of my surgeon, Mr Bose, and will assist with today's procedures. I sit next to her and start talking to her. I quickly realise she is a very dynamic person. She exudes passion and clearly knows where she is going in life. I tell her I plan to write a chapter on women in cardiac surgery and we agree to meet up and have a chat at a more convenient time.

The time has come to follow Dr Watson into the anaesthetic room. A wave of unease washes over me. The last time I saw a room like this I was the patient. This is the place I closed my eyes, stunned and afraid, on that afternoon in January 2017

Dr Watson and his assistant Damian explain what they are doing as they prepare to welcome our first patient. These two guys clearly have a unique working relationship as very few words are spoken, yet everything is positioned exactly where it should be.

A few moments later and our first patient walks into the room after being brought up from the ward by wheelchair. He is forty-nine years old and needs a replacement aortic valve. He is the gentleman I interviewed just the day before.

Yesterday he was very chatty, even upbeat, whilst telling me of his cardiac journey. Today, I barely recognise him. We don't make eye contact. His body language and facial expressions tell me this is a man full of anxiety, full of trepidation. He climbs onto the bed and leans back. I see his eyes and the piercing look of fear within them.

Dr Watson and Damian start to prepare the man to be anaesthetised. At this stage, I am overwhelmed by what I am seeing and can't understand some of the things that Dr Watson is telling me.

It takes about thirty minutes to prepare the patient.

Once anaesthetized, the patient is wheeled into the operating theatre which, for me, is like walking into the lion's den. About ten people are waiting, all but one in the same green scrubs as me. The patient is positioned under the lights, just as we see on TV. Only this is a real-life drama playing out in front of me.

Mr Bose addresses the assembled team and confirms what procedure is about to take place. He then asks everyone to introduce themselves, so we all know who's who and what their role and responsibilities are. When it comes to me, I tell them I am here to observe for a book I am about to write, so please don't ask me to do anything technical! One other observer is attending who is sitting at the far end of the theatre.

Mr Bose and Dr Watson begin positioning the TOE probe to visualise the patient's heart on a screen. I am flattered to be asked to look at the screen with them. They are looking to assess the function of the mitral valve. In this patient's case, it is possible that the mitral valve may also need replacing. To be honest, as somebody without the years of dedicated training, all I could see was a good reason to phone the television engineer. The screen to me looked like a melee of grey shadows, blurred images, and sporadic flashes of colour. I am told that blood flowing towards the probe is red whilst blood flowing away from it, is blue. If blood is observed flowing back through the valve what they call regurgitation, then they know the valve is not functioning correctly. It turns out the mitral valve looks good and won't require any treatment after all.

Now that everyone knows what is about to take place, the procedure gets underway. Most of the surgeons I have observed stand to the right of the patient while the anaesthetist stands at the head. The nursing team and perfusionist are on the periphery. Ms Hardman, who I had met moments earlier in the coffee room, is starting things off.

I am invited to stand alongside Dr Watson at the head of the patient. I get into position and look down. What I see is the chest of a human being. A human being that until a few moments ago, was wide awake and will have zero recollection of the next six hours in his life. I wonder if he will be as intrigued to find out what happened during that time as I am?

Now I don't know if this is normal for observers, as the other observer was sat well away from the operating table, but I was literally within three feet of the patient's chest - a similar distance to that of the surgeons and the anaesthetist. This was like having a ringside seat, inside the ring.

The procedure begins with a sternotomy. With all the confidence of a seasoned surgeon, Miss Hardman makes an incision down the centre of the chest. She works away with an instrument that cuts and cauterises the exposed tissues, so they don't bleed. Suddenly the sternum (breastbone) becomes visible. The next requirement is to saw down the centre of the breastbone so the two sides of the chest can be parted, granting access to the heart. It takes less than ten seconds to split the sternum.

As the two sides of the chest are clamped open, I get my first view of a real, beating human heart.

This would have been me on the table, my heart exposed just like this. I don't let on, but I am starting to get very emotional. I came here to find out what happened to me and the answer was unfolding right in front of me.

The next part of the procedure is truly remarkable.

Tony Walker told me that the performance of heart surgery is problematic for two reasons: firstly, the heart is full of blood, and secondly, the heart is always in motion. This is where the unsung heroes come into play. These heroes are called perfusionists. Perfusionists operate the heart-lung machine. This is a machine which takes over the functions of your heart and lungs, keeping oxygenated blood flowing to the rest of your body. The machine bypasses the heart and lungs so that no blood passes through them, enabling the surgeons to work their magic.

The heart also has to be stopped to allow for the valve to be fitted. This is called cardioplegia, another of the perfusionist's responsibilities.

As the surgeon calls for the pump to start, suddenly the heart monitor flatlines. I feel unnerved. Anywhere else in the hospital, the sound of the heart monitor flatlining would stir up a hive of frenetic activity. But not so in this environment. This is exactly what is required.

Mr Bose shows me the prosthetic valve which will replace the damaged one. Though it is biological – made from harvested animal cells – it looks synthetic to me. It is strange, a very unnatural white in colour. He also draws my attention to the damaged aortic valve. It looks a little like a deformed Mercedes-Benz badge. He points out where the 'leaflets' have become calcified, peeling back in such a way that they no longer make a seal. I am utterly transfixed, watching the deft hands of this practised master as he stitches in the replacement valve.

Gill Hardman is called a trainee surgeon, a name that seems totally inappropriate and rather patronising for the level of skill she is demonstrating. For me, she is an artist. In this moment art feels like the perfect metaphor for what these gifted surgeons do. They create masterpieces.

Approximately four hours later and the patient is all zipped up and ready to be taken to the CICU. Whilst Gill Hardman finishes off and does the paperwork, Mr Bose calls me out of theatre to follow him. He leads me to an office where he pulls up the angiogram images of the next patient. He explains to me what we can see and tells me the patient is having two coronary artery bypass grafts similar to what he performed on me the previous year. This operation involves bypassing an occluded (blocked) portion of the coronary arteries (the vessels which carry blood to the tissues of the heart itself).

By grafting a portion of the unblocked vessel to the affected artery, the surgeon can create a pathway for blood to flow without obstruction, bypassing the blocked area altogether. I try to look intelligent and ask a couple of questions I hope might make me sound as if I know what I am talking about.

Despite the morning's events, I still possess an appetite and we leave the office for lunch. The theatres are up on the second floor and the hospital shop is on the ground floor some distance away. Getting out of the theatre corridor is relatively easy. You just press a green button on the wall and the doors unlock for you. Getting back in, however, is not so straightforward.

Returning with my BLT, I learn that my visitor's pass is not programmed to open any doors. Now I am stuck in the outer corridor desperately trying to get someone on the inside to let me in. I begin to feel a little agitated, hoping I don't miss my chance to observe the second case. Eventually, someone stops by and I am asked to show my visitor's pass to regain entry. I must remember not to make that mistake again!

By the time I get back into the anaesthetic room, the next patient is already unconscious and almost ready to be wheeled into theatre. Once again registrar Gill Hardman is to take the lead under Amal Bose's watchful eye.

What I experience this afternoon continues to blow me away. It is incredible what can be done to the human body by these individuals who have practised and honed their skills over decades. This afternoon promises to be even more fascinating because, unlike this morning, the surgeons are going to do two coronary artery bypass grafts without stopping the heart.

The initial phase of the operation is similar to the morning. However, whilst Ms Hardman is opening up the chest a nurse is now cutting a long groove in the leg of the patient. This is to harvest a vessel to use for the two grafts required.

The big challenge with this operation is working with a beating heart. Clearly, it's much easier when the heart is stopped. With a beating heart, you have to work in pace with the heart's natural rhythm.

As before Mr Bose and Ms Hardman talk me through the procedure stage by stage. My absorption is interrupted by flashbacks. I still can't believe what I am seeing.

At one point, Amal cast a bemused glance my way, dryly suggesting, "You may see a lot clearer if you raise your headwear off your glasses." I thought the world had gone a little misty.

The procedure is successfully concluded in around three hours. Along with Ms Hardman and Dr Watson, I follow the patient into the CICU unit.

The patient is still unconscious and would remain that way until the intensive care anaesthetist decides he is ready to be brought around.

I am chatting with Gill Hardman when Dr Helen Saunders, a consultant cardiac anaesthetist and divisional director, arrives and asks me how my day had gone. I tell her it was an amazing experience and how impressed I am with the team and the way they seamlessly worked as a unit. At this point, however, I was so exhausted I had forgotten Ms Hardman's name, could not remember the word "perfusionist", and called Dr Dale Watson "David". After some eight hours in theatre, my brain was waving a white flag and all I had done was stand and watch. Mr Bose, Miss Hardman, and Dr Watson had spent the same time in intense concentration, with the responsibility of two people's lives in their hands. I am in awe of how these guys can do this - their mental and physical fortitude is *superhuman.*

Ms Hardman and Mr Bose were on call that evening, and an emergency had just arrived which required urgent surgical intervention. Another theatre session could feasibly extend their day past eighteen hours, perhaps longer still.

Dr Saunders, who was not on call, and her fellow anaesthetists, including Dr Watson had collectively decided to go out for dinner that night. Me on the other hand, I was only fit for one thing, bed.

It's the day after my first theatre experience and I'm embarrassed to say that tears are streaming down my face as I write up my first day in theatre. The whole experience meant a great deal to me. I could now understand what had happened during my own procedure. The sheer enormity of it. My experience gave me some much-needed closure and helped me realise the severity of the trauma my body had endured.

I found my first visit to theatre inspiring. I had seen my surgeon, Mr Bose, in action and it had opened my eyes. I also learned he has a wicked sense of humour when he works. Most of the staff in theatre wear the supplied NHS headwear. Mr Bose, on the other hand, has his own. It's black and has the words *The Legend Lives* all over it. One day I will drum up the courage to ask him who the 'Legend' is, although I think I have a pretty good idea.

Mr Bose is clearly a surgeon at the very top of his game, the equivalent of Cristiano Ronaldo or Roger Federer. He exudes an air of total control. His confidence and his ability to cope calmly is incredible to watch.

I stop writing for a moment and slouch back in my chair, giving myself a few moments to appreciate how privileged I am to have had this experience.

It's now a week following my first day in cardiac theatres and I am again taking a trip down to Blackpool. Today I want to meet the patients as they arrive and get checked in at same-day admission. Patients are either admitted the day before surgery to stay the night on the ward or are called in on the morning of their procedure, known as same-day admissions. I am interested to witness their emotional states and compare them to how I felt going through the same process.

An NHS national report called "GIRFT" (Get It Right First Time) had recently been published and highly commended the Lancashire Cardiac Centre for its successful practice of same-day admissions. More than 65% of elective surgery at Blackpool is based on same-day admissions, the envy of other cardiac centres. Same-day admissions help to alleviate the pressure of bed shortages and ensure that capacity is utilised efficiently.

The first admissions would arrive around seven o'clock, so I rise at four-thirty, eager as ever to set off with time to spare. Sunlight is just beginning to spill across the fells as I leave our remote Cumbrian cottage, trying not to set the dogs off barking. The only sounds I can hear are the sheep on the hills as they welcomed yet another day in paradise with their incessant bleating.

Once again, I drive carefully down our bumpy track past our two Shetland ponies who were munching on grass in the paddock. One gazed up as if to say, "where the hell are you going at this time of the day?"

I arrive with enough time to park up and make my way to the Same-Day Admissions Unit. On arrival, Dawn and Tracy, who run the unit, are already well into setting up for the first patient's arrival. Today, there are seven coming in for procedures.

Dawn has been doing this job for many years and appreciates the range of emotions people can be experiencing when they arrive. I remember Dawn from when I came in. She had looked after me, checking my details and taking my blood pressure. I remember she asked me if I was wearing nail varnish. Dawn saw my surprise at this question and hastily qualified it with "this is Blackpool, the gay capital of the north."

The first person to arrive today is John. John had already been asked if I could speak with him prior to going in and he had kindly agreed. John is Irish, aged eighty-three, and is here to have a nodule on his lung biopsied to see if it is malignant. John understandably looks and sounds very apprehensive. Today his world may be turned upside down by the words no one ever wants to hear.

The second person to arrive is Ian, an ex-army man and the opposite end of the emotional spectrum to John. I don't have prior consent to talk to Ian. As he walks in Dawn introduces me and I say I am happy to leave. Ian is full of bravado (or is this his way of dealing with a very stressful situation?) He assures me I can stay and tells me he is not worried about what's ahead. "What will be will be" he exclaims admirably. Ian is asked if he is wearing nail varnish. "You must be joking," he says. After some laughter, Ian leaves the room to be shaved and that's the last I see of him.

While we wait for our next patient, Dawn and Tracy tell me the story of a previous patient. He was a builder, a tall man (over six foot) and the epitome of media projected masculinity. When it came to the nail varnish question, he suddenly became very flustered, turning bright red in the face. The ladies explained the reason why nail varnish could not be tolerated. He sheepishly owned up to having nail varnish on his toes and put it down to messing around with his young daughter the night before, Dawn concluded that the jury was still out on that one.

The third patient I see is a woman, let's call her Helen. Helen looks very nervous. Her voice is quiet and trembling with apprehension. Another woman appears. I say hello and she introduces herself as Julie from the Alcohol Awareness Programme. Curious, I ask her what that is, and she explains.

As mentioned earlier, patients visit the hospital before the procedure for a pre-operative assessment. Anything from a fortnight to a day prior to your procedure you come into the hospital to have a series of investigations which include blood, swabs, as well as a review with an anaesthetist. These results are all required by the theatre team before surgery can take place. One question they ask is, "How many units of alcohol a week do you consume?" Apparently, but not surprisingly, a large majority of us lie and reduce our real intake to something that sounds acceptable. Helen's alcohol consumption had raised a few alarm bells and therefore Julie was asked to come in to have a discrete chat with her.

I asked Julie how big a problem alcohol was. She said it is much bigger than you think. Many people have a glass of wine or a can of beer when they get home to relieve the stress of the working day. They might have one more over dinner and maybe even a nightcap before bed. Do this seven days a week and you're well over the recommended limit. Go to the pub a few times a week and you are significantly over the proposed weekly limit. Drink has a massive effect on recovery and alcohol dependency can play a major role in whether surgery is offered or not.

As I am talking to Julie, Dr Saunders arrives to escort me up to theatre. Today she is working in her capacity as a consultant anaesthetist alongside Mr Bittar, the surgeon I am going to observe.

John, the patient I met in same-day admissions earlier, arrives in the anaesthetic room looking extremely nervous. In a few hours, he will know if his lung nodule is malignant or not.

Before Dr Saunders starts to anaesthetise him, Mr Bittar comes in to explain to John exactly what the plan is and what the possibilities are, subject to the results of the biopsy.

It doesn't take long before Dr Saunders has worked her magic and the patient is ready to be taken in. Stepping into the operating theatre this time I feel a bit more comfortable on this visit and more aware of my surroundings. When I was watching heart surgery the previous week the chest was opened up, so the heart became visible, but the lungs were still inaccessible. I wondered how surgeons got to the lungs.

With some careful manoeuvring and the use of some clever airbags the patient is positioned on his side. The lung which requires intervention, right or left, determines which side the patient is turned onto.

I am here today to witness some minimally invasive surgery. The whole operation is going to be carried out through three small incisions made on the side of the breastbone allowing access between the ribs. Minimally invasive surgery demands a whole new set of skills. Some surgeons have been unable to make the transition owing to the level of hand-to-eye coordination demanded.

The surgical site is projected onto a large screen which is connected to a camera on a probe inserted through one of the three incisions. The lights are turned off so that the images on the screen can be viewed with maximum clarity. The image is nothing short of stunning, displayed in high-definition 3D. The surgeons wear 3D glasses which give them an incredible representation of size, depth, and realism. I was fortunate to be given a pair as well. The 3D image of a living human's lung is something I will never forget.

Working in tandem with his registrar, Mr Bittar uses a series of different instruments that enter the body via the three incisions made in the chest wall earlier. Mr Bittar is looking at the screen which is displaying 3D images from the camera positioned around the lungs. Mr Bittar carefully manoeuvres the instruments to remove the nodule from the lung. To understand what I am seeing, imagine using an absurdly long-handled knife and fork to eat your dinner, only your dinner is inside a box with a pair of holes in one side.

Mr Bittar, demonstrating impeccable skill and the most amazing hand-to-eye coordination, has now located and cut the nodule out. He inserts what looks like a little plastic bag through one of the holes and places the nodule inside it. This is swiftly taken away to the pathology labs where it will be analysed to confirm whether or not it is malignant. I am told this process will take about 40 minutes.

While we wait, Mr Bittar continues to plan his course of action should the prognosis be a poor one. If that turns out to be the case, then the plan is to take away the top portion of the lung and hopefully cancer with it.

I watch in amazement and ask myself how some human beings can be this talented and knowledgeable. I am a big fan of Eggheads, the BBC 2 quiz programme. One of the Eggheads is a man called Kevin Ashman. Kevin seems to know everything about everything. All of the Eggheads are incredibly knowledgeable, but Kevin appears to be on a different planet. How is it possible to obtain such vast knowledge when there are only 24 hours in a day? Watching Mr Bittar perform and appreciating the general knowledge Kevin Ashman has on Eggheads does nothing for my self-esteem as I realise the intellectual gulf there is between us!

Forty minutes elapse and someone is sent to the lab for the results. I can feel the tension in the room. It's at least five more minutes before the news arrives. The nodule is… *non*-malignant. There is a big sigh of relief in the theatre. Mr Bittar tells his registrar to close the patient back up again before taking off his gown and gloves and disappearing out of the theatre.

The patient remains in the hands of Dr Saunders who is responsible for his safety, keeping him sedated until he is ready to be transferred.

I take a moment to imagine the incredible relief John and his family will feel when they get the good news. A few hours ago, they were preparing to hear the worst. Now, John has his life back. He has been reborn.

Dr Saunders and the rest of the team move John onto his back and then onto a bed to be transferred to CICU where I will catch up with him later. We break for an early lunch, but Dr Saunders and Mr Bittar ask for the next patient to be readied for theatre.

I was busy with my research on the internet when I just happened to come across 'The World's Most Luxurious Homes.' It was an inside look into celebrity 'cribs' and the lifestyles of the rich and famous. Later, I went into the lounge to watch the evening news. First up was Syria and the continued devastation of that once beautiful country and its people. It showed how families were living in bombed-out towns with little infrastructure and nowhere to call home.

This really brought home how life is so full of extremes. Many celebrities worry about luxurious homes, holiday villas, and private jets. All the Syrians would like is not to wake up to the screaming sound of aircraft overhead, followed by total carnage.

Mr Bittar, one of the cardiothoracic surgeons I have been privileged to observe and get to know, is Syrian and some of his family still live there.

Consultant Cardiac Surgeon Mr Bittar – His story
Nadil Bittar He was born in 1968 in the northern Syrian town of Idlib. What emotional stress you must be under living away from it, but having family still there, living in a town that is the stronghold of ISIS. How do you communicate when most of the infrastructure has been shattered?

Nadil's mother and father were teachers. He has four brothers and four sisters. Six of them are medical doctors, one is an engineer and one is an economist.

He always wanted to be a doctor and followed his older brothers and sisters into medical school.

He decided to come to the UK in March 1996. When he arrived, his English wasn't brilliant so the first few months were interesting, to say the least. He went to night school and within a few months, his English improved dramatically.

He started as a house officer, then did spells in casualty and general surgery just to comply with the regulations to sit the exams. Between 1996 and 1999, he studied and qualified in cardiothoracic and general surgery.

He did some cardiothoracic research at Wythenshawe Hospital, Greater Manchester. At that time, the waiting list for a procedure was eighteen months to two years. The government made cardiothoracic a priority and so more surgeons were required, and Mr Bittar became a training member (this is something you must acquire if you want to become a surgeon and apply for jobs).

He took on a locum position at Blackpool before becoming a valuable permanent member of the team.

I asked him what he does when he is not in theatre and his response was quite enlightening. Like many of the people I have interviewed, Nadil agrees that the job has a habit of consuming you 24/7. That's why there are only three-hundred people who do it out of sixty-six million in the country. Even when on holiday, he is answering emails and checking on patients. So, you have to create a distraction from it. His release is doing adventurous things to raise funding for charities.

He has run the London marathon in six hours and twenty-nine minutes.

When I return to theatre after lunch, Dr Saunders has already anaesthetised the next patient. She tells me the patient was shaking with fear when he came in. I ask Dr Saunders if part of her formal training included sessions on how to manage the spectrum of patient emotions. She tells me that there is much more formal input now, but her ability came from experience. Throughout this second case, I spend more time talking to Dr Saunders. I want to find out a bit more about her journey and why she wanted to become an anaesthetist. On the face of it, Dr Saunders appears to be a very unassuming individual. Yet at 6 o'clock that morning she was doing a gym session of boxing training, at the weekend she was planning to do a triathlon.

I am scheduled to watch three procedures that day but unfortunately, the bed shortage felt across the NHS, reared its ugly head. Surgeons cannot undertake procedures unless there is a CICU bed for the patient confirmed in advance. There are 20 CICU beds in the cardiac centre. Everyone who has major cardiothoracic surgery recovers in CICU immediately after the operation. Patients already on CICU can only be moved to the wards when they are fit enough. The previous day saw a large number of emergency cases which had a big impact on capacity.

Bed shortages in other areas of the hospital also make an impact. As is publically documented, general hospital admissions spike during the winter. In order to cope with the additional pressure, a number of beds on the cardiac ward have been allocated to medical patients. When the ward is full, it means that patients on CICU who are ready to be moved down have to stay until a bed on the ward become available.

The team holds out until 2:00pm before being told there definitely wouldn't be a bed for Mr Bittar's third patient. At this point, there are several people downstairs who are expecting surgery today.

Having your procedure cancelled at the last moment can be emotionally shattering for the patient and their family. Just imagine the stress of arriving at the hospital, going through all the checks, and waiting for hours only to be told moments before its due to happen it's been cancelled. In preparation for general anaesthetic patients also have to be starved for a number of hours before the procedure. You may have stayed overnight, if you live some distance away, your family may have taken time off work to be with you. This is one of the toughest situations for the surgeons as they are the people who generally have to go and deliver the devastating news to people who are apprehensive, tired, and hungry. The patient reaction varies but the disappointment is universal.

Dr Saunders and I go to see the patients who had their surgery earlier. Both of them are still very drowsy and are not in a fit state for a chat. However, both say they have severe pain in their shoulder. This apparently is not uncommon after lung surgery. With no further cases going ahead, I thank the team for their time and head back home.

Looking back at my first two days in theatre has left me with many questions and many insights. It has been an amazing experience and makes me appreciate the dedication, enthusiasm, and the incredible level of skill these professionals demonstrate.

Driving home, I begin to reflect how today has changed over a period of a few hours. I think about all of those people's journeys, including my own, that have taken a detour via the Lancashire Cardiac Centre.

Spending a day with very poorly people has given me focus. There's a well-known saying, 'health is wealth'. As you get older, the quote becomes increasingly relevant. Having all the money in the world is pointless unless you have the health to enjoy it. As I drive off the main road and onto the single-track lane with views over the Lakeland fells, I am filled with appreciation for where I live and how precious life is.

Another week has gone by and I am heading back to Blackpool. This time I am going to the catheter labs to watch a cardiologist perform a catheter ablation. This is a minimally invasive procedure to address arrhythmias which have not responded to medication management. A catheter is inserted into the groin and very skillfully manoeuvred up into the heart. Once it is in place, the consultant can stop the electrical impulses that are causing the problem. Today it is going to be done by Dr Chalil, a consultant cardiologist and electrophysiologist:

I had the pleasure of interviewing Dr Chalil.

Consultant Cardiologist Dr Chalil - His story

I meet Shajil in the corridor outside his office, though not for the first time, as I am one of his patients. A considerate man, he wants to know how my health is. We discuss my condition briefly before sitting down. Knowing the doctor's time is precious I switch on my mini tape recorder and am ready to begin.

The first thing I'm eager to find out is the point in his life when he realised he wanted to be a doctor. He tells me he knew when he was just five years old. His dad's friend was a paediatrician whom he admired greatly. His aunt was also a doctor. A young Shajil was amazed at what a difference these people could make to the lives of others. From then on, he never wanted to be anything else.

At the age of nine, he changed schools due to his father's work. The principal of the school asked him what he wanted to be, and he told him he wanted to be a doctor. The principal asked how could he be so sure he would be a doctor? He openly admits that he was a pretty confident young man and when he got into medical school, he wrote to the principal to tell him he was on his way to becoming that doctor.

He did his medical degree in Madras, known now as Chennai, in India. It was at medical school that he realised paediatrics was not for him. By the time he came to Britain in 2000, he was certain he wanted to do his MRCP and go on to be a cardiologist. In those days, training posts were much rarer than they are now. Competition for places was fierce. To get a training number, which you need to become a consultant, was very difficult.

He worked with a consultant called Dr Salker in Eastbourne. His passion for cardiology was realised thanks to some great mentors who guided him and told him to work hard. It was in Eastbourne where Dr Chalil did his first pacemaker and his first angiogram.

I want to know what he considers to be the qualities of a fine doctor. His reply, "To be a good human being, that is the cornerstone you start from."

As the conversation went on, Dr Chalil offered me an insight into his working life. He says the last few days, his working day had started at 7am and he had not got home much earlier than 9pm The extra hours are all unpaid but as long as a patient is in need of his help then he will make himself available. He feels this is his duty and why he does what he does. He made it very clear that you don't become a doctor for a nice life. If that's your motivation, then you should be in another profession. Being a doctor is not a nine-to-five job.

He does, however, have a family. A wife who is a GP and a daughter who is about to become a teenager. His daughter, fortunately, understands that mum and dad have demanding jobs and that's why the previous *weekend's family plans were shelved. Even though she is witness to the stresses and strains of the profession, his daughter has also decided she wants to become a doctor.*

It's not just the hours that are demanding. For every procedure that takes place, there is a chance of complications or an undesirable outcome. On the rare occasion when it happens, then you question yourself a thousand times. Doctors are only human and sometimes, the public can forget that.

The conversation moves to teamwork. I ask how many teams does he think he is in? He highlights that he is part of the team that is close to him; registrars, secretaries, healthcare assistants, nurses, the people he interacts with daily. But he shows an incredible sensitivity to the bigger picture. He appreciates that there is a huge number of team members he doesn't see, whose names he doesn't know, but who deliver critical elements of the service that enable him to do what he does. Receptionists, the volunteers who help people find his clinic, porters, the lab technicians. He is part of their team too. Dr Chalil believes that the success of the cardiac centre depends not just on one person but the many people who fulfil their roles every day.

As I enter the catheter lab, Dr Chalil is at the other end of the corridor. I watch him for a few moments. He is wearing what looks like a long bulletproof vest. I can see from his demeanour that he is totally focused, in the zone. He hasn't noticed me loitering yet. We eventually make eye contact and he begins to approach. We take a moment to exchange pleasantries and he tells me I am about to observe his second patient of the day. It's barely 9:00am and he has already completed one procedure.

He leads me into the waiting room where his next patient is waiting with his wife. I introduce myself to them and thank them both for consenting me to watch the procedure. Our conversation is interrupted as I am asked to go and get my own bulletproof vest on before entering the lab. I learn that the procedure is under x-ray and the vests are to protect against radiation.

The next time I see the patient, he is under the lights. Shajil is standing over him and ready to begin. I watch in amazement. The next one and a half hours I stand behind a lead glass barrier watching a 3D map of the patient's heart on-screen. He is looking to identify where the electrical signals responsible for the arrhythmia are coming from. It is delicate work and I am once again humbled by the incredible display of skill I am witnessing.

Once the procedure is completed, I have a brief chat with Dr Chalil about the procedures, thanking him for allowing me the opportunity to witness yet another amazing day.

Heart surgery has come a very long way over the last fifty years, and that's down to very clever people who think life is all about pushing the boundaries. Surgeons like Christian Barnard, a South African surgeon who performed the first successful heart transplant in 1967. His pioneering approach shows what the human spirit is capable of. Such remarkable things can only result from exploration, and the will to further the frontiers of possibility.

Another surgeon who was there in the early days of pioneering heart surgery is Mr Andrew Duncan. After chasing him through his secretary Amanda, I was privileged to get an interview with him.

Mr Duncan, or as I would like to affectionally call him, 'The Grand Master', heads up the cardiac department at the Blackpool Victoria Hospital and has a vast depth of knowledge and experience of all things surgical. I was told by Amanda that Mr Duncan only had a thirty-minute slot to offer.

Consultant Cardiac Surgeon Mr Duncan - His story

In his early years, Andrew Duncan remembers being interested in the sciences when he was in school and taking a pig's heart into a lesson to talk about how a heart worked. That's what he likes about cardiac surgery; you have to be a scientist, a physiologist, a doctor as well as a technician. You have to bring a whole ream of skills together to make it work, including the ability to work with a diversely skilled team of people.

As a student, he spent three weeks in the Cardiothoracic department and really got excited by the skill of the individuals, their dedication and how mentally tough they were. But then, they had to be, because back then, people would die much more frequently than they do today. Bleeding, trauma and complications were part of the days' work.

Mr Duncan felt that the special passion that members of the cardiac teams appear to have, is because of the enormity of the situation. You do literally have someone's life in your hands. When it goes wrong, it's you that has to resolve it. He continues to say the patient's family is just down the corridor waiting for you to come out and give them the good news. Unfortunately, although very rare; it does go wrong and it does sit firmly with you. That is an incredibly tough part of the job and one you can or can't do.

As far as feeling a rollercoaster of emotions when he's in theatre, his response was, "For the first fifteen years, I was very nervous about getting it right but in the last seven years, I have grown dramatically and become much more confident in my own ability."' Now he has passed the 10,000 surgical procedures he calls himself 'unconsciously competent,' where he feels in control of any situation.

On teamwork, he felt that most procedures have a process and protocols, the individuals know the stages and are, therefore, ready to play their part. As an example, when Mr Duncan is ready to join the two ends of a vein together, the scrub nurse would know that he will need a stitch.

As we are talking, the phone rings and as if to highlight that the Grand Master is human like the rest of us, the person on the end of the line is his son enquiring where the jump leads are. It would seem even Grand Masters have issues with car batteries going flat. As the conversation continues, I indicate that I will leave so he can have a private conversation, but he waves his finger for me to sit back down.

We have a little chuckle about life getting in the way. He explains his vision of a department that is completely 'patient-focused' and working as a team to deliver the best journey and outcome possible. To achieve this, it is important that the department is on its own continuous improvement journey. The department does do some simulation training; however, he says nothing can coach a new scrub nurse better than a real situation. Over the years, with a small group of colleagues, Mr Duncan has introduced many processes and protocols that are now being replicated by other surgeons around the world, which must be the highest form of recognition. He highlights that he does most of his graft procedures 'off-pump' which means the two people he works closest to are the scrub nurse and the anaesthetist. The three of them must have a clear understanding, even if it isn't telepathy.

Andrew pioneered 'off-pump' surgery in 2000. He openly admits that at the time, it was terrifying but now it's second nature. He explains that 'on-pump' you are against time, as the heart is being starved of blood. 'Off-pump', there is less rush, as the heart is being naturally supplied with blood. It does, however, mean you have to have meticulous planning in that the heart needs to be in a particular position. Getting everything right is a challenge, one he took on with enthusiasm.

I am now some thirty minutes into the interview. It is very clear Mr Duncan loves a challenge. If 'off-pump' was a challenge, then developing a skill set to undertake minimal invasive lung surgery was also embraced with the commitment you would expect from a Grand Master. Most surgeons doing this procedure do it with the help of a large 3D screen that gives a real view of the size and depth of the lungs. He does his procedures in 2D saying his brain can interpret size and depth from the 2D images.

I am intrigued to know how and more importantly, why he can do it in 2D, when most surgeons need 3D. He continues to say that although every surgeon has a level of skill, it's more about how the brain is wired. Some people can do it, and some can't. I'm fascinated with how you learn to do procedures that clearly need an understanding of size and shape in 2D. I expected a very intellectual response. The reality was very different. "I forgot to switch the 3D function on and did the whole procedure in 2D before realizing," was his response!

The phone rings again. This time, it's Mr Duncan's wife, still trying to resolve the car issue. I observe that these consultants are no different from any of us in family issues. I will leave you to interpret that comment in your own way.

I asked which era he felt was the best to learn to be a surgeon, the early days or now? He chose the early days with much enthusiasm, the reason being, he learnt to operate on anything inside the chest. Today's surgeons are becoming very specialised.

I am interested to know how much cardiac surgery has changed over the period, considering that it is a newish discipline. Mr Duncan explains what has happened is things have got better and more refined. For example, the by-pass machines are now very sophisticated compared to the early versions, stitches are better, basically, procedures have not changed too much but the way they are undertaken, and the technology and equipment has improved enormously.

He is fascinated by the history of cardiac surgery and explains to me that it all started with the early tuberculosis surgeons who would travel around performing operations on people and losing many through bleeding but just kept on going, perfecting the procedure. When tuberculosis died out, they moved across to the heart but had no experience so they would end up cooling the heart down in an ice bath which gave them about eight minutes to complete the surgery. Then they would end up sewing the wrong bits together.

He remembers looking at the theatre book for the 1960s in Edinburgh and every third patient died. But then on reflection, many of these had irreversible congenital heart disease where it was discovered too late. There were no valve procedures back then because replacement valves weren't available.

Sitting with the Grand Master listening to his vast depth of stories is like having an audience with the incredible raconteur, Peter Ustinov. The stories just kept coming. Again, we go back to the early days of cardiac surgery and a story of an American surgeon whose first seven patients died. The surgeon decided that emotionally, he could no longer continue. That was until a cardiologist called him and said he must do an operation. He did, the patient survived, and the surgeon went on to be one of the most celebrated in America. What strength of character to have that mortality rate and still keep going... amazing!

Again, the stories keep on coming. He recalls when he started doing heart surgery back in 1987, in one week alone they had five deaths in the intensive care unit. How different that is to now when a fatality from heart surgery is extremely rare. From where I sit, that comes from the pioneers like Andrew who understood what was possible, it just needed refining. Now the success rate is around 98% and the cases now being undertaken are much more complex and on much older patients.

Success is now expected. That's not arrogance, it's just all the surgeons are so highly trained, accomplished and have many successful procedures and experience to draw from.

As head of the department, he has created the motto, 'If it looks nice, it's right.' It's all about technical perfection.

He owns up to being a perfectionist, and then we laugh out loud as when we look around his office, there are files everywhere. He quickly defends the situation by saying that perfection is not required in all areas.

I realise I have been in his company for over an hour now and don't want to overstay my welcome, so I want to get his view on the future of cardiac surgery and the burning question for me is why, in this technological age, isn't there a replacement heart? I am the proud owner of an artificial right knee, so why not a heart?

With incredible new composites and the technology that we have today, why haven't we been able to develop an artificial heart? I am told huge research has gone into this area, but the artificial heart always created complications, like the body rejecting them and parts failing. Mr Duncan believes the best route is to develop animal hearts that could be transferred. That said, there are lots of viral genes in an animal heart that can cause tumours and rejection.

The human heart is a masterpiece of human engineering. It never stops, it beats roughly 70 beats a minute, 100,000 times a day and does that on average for 70-90 years. When you think of all the hearts in a world of some eight billion people, they have an incredible safety record. Nothing man-made can get close to that reliability.

Our thirty-minute planned interview has now turned into ninety, I could spend the same time again, as it has been such an entertaining and incredibly informative time.

Andrew Duncan is 'old school.' By that, I mean his experience has taken place over the decades. He has been part of heart surgery development from its infancy. Modern-day surgeons tend to specialise in one area and master that procedure.

If you think of career success as a triangle and you want to reach the pinnacle of success, then your knowledge base has to be as wide as possible to give you the stability to get to the highest point. Mr Duncan probably doesn't use all his knowledge base but it's there if the situation requires it.

Over the course of my research for this book, I was lucky to have many more experiences like the ones in this chapter. I have been left with a deep appreciation for just how lucky we are, that there are such human beings in the world to care for us when we hear those words we never want to hear.

Reader Question

I have had many dramas in my life, yet in reality, most of them didn't matter.

What really matters to you in your life?

Chapter 5

What a Performance!

"The most important thing is to live a fabulous life. As long as it's fabulous, I don't care how long it is."

When you think of creative performance, you probably think of music or a theatrical play. In both, there is usually a lead figure, whether it be a lead singer in a band or a star performer in a West End production. This is perhaps not so different from the operating theatre. In fact, in days gone by, operations were also performed before an audience of students in tiered seating, hence the name operating theatre.

Sport is often the go-to metaphor for thinking about business, teamwork, communication, and success. There is a whole business sector of ex-sporting celebrities using their experience to present winning, teamwork, and leadership methodology to the corporate world. However, I feel such metaphors are overused and inappropriate, being as they are based on winning and losing. Losing is not an acceptable end result in a cardiac theatre.

Throughout the course of writing this book, it became clear to me that cardiac surgery could not fit into this sporting arena. Cardiac surgery is better seen as the advancement of *art*. It is a triumph over adversity rather than a triumph over the competition.

I have always found it fascinating how so many people set out on a career path but how few reach the top. Think of a mountain with everyone starting at the base, whether they be a lead guitarist, actor, or consultant surgeon. As the climb begins people start to fall by the wayside. "It's too hard." "It's not what I thought it would be." As we approach the summit, major obstacles stand in our way, obstacles which will challenge every sinew of our body and soul. The terrain is there as if to declare "only the strongest will succeed". Look at any profession: there are only a few at the very top. In the UK, there are a mere three-hundred consultant heart surgeons.

During my work with elite professional football teams, I would see some amazing players during training. They would show incredible skill five days a week. But on a Saturday in front of forty thousand spectators, some just could not perform. I wonder how many great singers, actors, and budding surgeons' careers have been cut short for the same reasons?

But a musician, actor, or surgeon cannot deliver a world-class performance on their own. In a West End production, you have the main character, the one that most of the attention is focused on, and then you have their co-stars. There are even more actors playing less prominent roles and also those who only have a short appearance or appear as extras. In a rock band, you have the singer who is typically the guy or gal upfront. You then have the lead guitarist, bassist, and drummer. Each of them must fulfil their roles in order for the performance to succeed. The singer may receive the greater share of adulation but if the drummer fails to keep the beat on track, then the whole performance falls apart. Similarly, while much of the focus is laid on the consultant surgeon, they cannot achieve success without their supporting cast. They rely on the anaesthetist, scrub nurse, registrar, perfusionist, nursing staff, and so on. Everybody has an essential part to play.

Before undertaking this journey, I would expect the public perception of what an anaesthetist does to be similar to mine. I thought all they did was give you an injection to put you to sleep and that was it, job done. How wrong could I be? Anaesthetists are extremely clever people. Their knowledge of anatomy and physiology is nothing short of staggering. Where the surgeon is a 'master of repairing' the heart, the anaesthetist is the oracle for everything else.

Their contact with the patient will start at the pre-operative assessment. This takes place in the hospital about a week to a fortnight before the procedure. A number of investigations are carried out including a range of blood tests, swabs, and a chest x-ray. The anaesthetist will want to know many pieces of information including how much you weigh, if you smoke or drink and what medications you take. This is to help them determine how you will take to anaesthesia and whether there are likely to be any complications either in theatre or during your recovery.

On the morning of your admission, it's the anaesthetist you will most likely see before your procedure. They need to check your circumstances have not changed and may recap on the procedure you are about to undertake to make sure you understand the situation. The next time you see them will be in the anaesthetic room.

During the procedure, as the surgeon concentrates on fixing the heart, the anaesthetist is responsible for monitoring all our vital signs. On screens all around the theatre, you can see readouts of the patient's heart rate, blood pressure etc etc. The heart itself is visualised by means of a transoesophageal echocardiogram probe (TOE) for which the anaesthetist is also responsible. Cardiac procedures can take a long time, sometimes much longer than anticipated, so the anaesthetist has to maintain an open dialogue with the surgeon to keep the patient sedated should the procedure last longer than expected.

Once the patient is transferred from theatre to the CICU, they become the responsibility of the anaesthetist on the ward and the numerous dedicated professionals that work on the ward across the shift pattern. An anaesthetist is always scheduled to work on intensive care to check on the patients.

Dr Noel Gavin has been a consultant anaesthetist at Blackpool for many years. I have been privileged to have witnessed Dr Gavin at work a number of times throughout my numerous visits to the department. I wanted to know more about the life of an anaesthetist, so I asked Dr Gavin for an interview. Happily, he agreed.

Consultant Anaesthetist Dr Gavin - His story
Irish and with a fantastic sense of humour, tongue very firmly in cheek, Noel Gavin claims to be, 'The world's

second-best anaesthetist.' When you ask him why only second best, he smiles and says, "There must be someone better." He is a very affable chap and, like many of his colleagues, he commits some of his personal time to charity work. Amal Bose has given his time to operate on children in India, Nadil Bittar raises huge amounts of money through bike rides, and Noel Gavin, for his part, works with a charity based in New Zealand through which he supports surgical procedures on remote Pacific Islands.

He graduated from medical school in Dublin in 1980. His initial plan was to become a cardiologist, but he had fallen out of love with the idea. During his time in the hospital, he got involved with intensive care. A lot of people in intensive care are anaesthetists. A year and a half spent in the midlands lead to a move to Wythenshawe Hospital in Greater Manchester via Perth, Australia. In time, he secured a consultant anaesthetist post at the Blackpool Victoria Hospital.

At that time, during the early nineties, the hospital in Blackpool was only doing around 250 cardiac procedures a year, but moving with the politics of the time, the chief executive decided the department needed to be expanded. Dr Gavin was instrumental in helping the department expand throughout this period.

I always find it interesting to discover why people go into their profession, so I ask Dr Gavin what he liked most of all about anaesthetics. From the smiley chap he is, his facial expression changed dramatically, and he suddenly became very serious. He recalled that from his medical student days, he had always had a fascination with the heart. He explained that his role as a cardiac anaesthetist is to look after the patient before the procedure, during the procedure, and to return the patient to a stable condition after the procedure. He tells *me that on the days when he is in theatre, he can concentrate 100% on his one or two patients and give them the very best experience possible.*

Dr Gavin informed me that when caring for older patients, the greatest challenge tends to be in the post-operative period. Older patients typically take longer to wake up and are at greater risk of complications such as developing infections and cognitive impairment. In fact, back in the eighties at Wythenshawe, they never offered a procedure to anyone over sixty-five years-of-age, as the risk was considered too great. Now Blackpool has successfully operated on patients over one hundred years-of-age. On hearing this, I felt compelled to ask a very controversial question: was it the best use of NHS funding to operate on people that old? Dr Gavin's response was, "As a consultant, I don't make the rules. If a patient is fit enough to cope with the procedure, then we operate." He added, "If it were your mum or dad, would you want them to receive the treatment?"

Yet despite the age of operable patients going up, the mortality rate has come significantly down. In the early days of cardiac surgery, there simply wasn't the abundance of knowledge we possess today and so there were very few protocols in place. The pioneers had to proceed by trial and error before arriving at a number of established techniques. Advancements in technology have also contributed to better outcomes, enabling pharmaceutical companies to refine the anaesthetic toolkit. This has resulted in fewer long-term effects on the body and a shorter reaction time than the earlier drugs. I am intrigued to learn that Noel believes today's surgeons are better than the surgeons of the nineties. I would love to get him and Andrew Duncan together, as he firmly believes the opposite.

In a rock band, when on stage, the drummer normally sits towards the back. Just so, as the rhythm they keep is the background, the foundation, of the whole performance. This is not at all dissimilar to the role which a perfusionist plays in cardiac surgery. As we found out earlier, the perfusionist is the person who looks after the bypass machine, the machine that bypasses the function of the patient's heart and lungs.

The machine itself actually does bear some resemblance to a drum kit. It has a number of cylinders that could be perceived as snare drums or tom-toms as well as a few screens suspended just above them, looking a little like cymbals. The perfusionist sits behind these just like a drummer. And just like a drummer, the perfusionist takes care of the foundation: the rhythm of the patients' life is in their hands.

It is the perfusionist's responsibility to deliver the drugs that stop and restart the heart as well as the drugs which prevent blood from clotting inside the machine. The perfusionist monitors the patient's various physiological parameters and makes appropriate pharmacological and thermal adjustments to maintain an optimal state. Much of their time is spent in cardiac theatres but now they may also find their responsibilities extending to areas such as the intensive care unit and catheter labs. To perform these tasks, a perfusionist must have a thorough understanding of both the respiratory and circulatory system and be able to operate complex equipment.

Today, I am meeting Andy Heggie, head of cardiac perfusion at Blackpool Victoria Hospital. He has organised a meeting with three members of his team to help me try and understand a bit more about the role of the perfusionist and how they got into the profession. We agreed to meet at around 9:00am and so, as always, I give myself plenty of time to make the trip and to collate thoughts and questions about what I need from the meeting.

Andy has been a healthcare professional for more than thirty-five years. He now holds the proud distinction of being the Chairman of the 'Society of Clinical Perfusion Scientists' and is an examiner for the society assessing junior perfusionists. Andy originally trained in cardiology. However, he happened to be observing in a cardiac theatre one day and saw a bypass machine in operation. From that moment Andy knew he would do whatever was necessary to become a perfusionist.

I have witnessed Andy at work on a number of occasions and it struck me how laid back he seems. That said there is no doubt Andy is totally in control of any situation and dedicated to the work he does. His leadership and insight inspire his team to set the bar high on every element of their work.

Now unless you had the misfortune of being one of the 30,000 people in the UK who have elective heart surgery each year, then you probably wouldn't have a clue what a perfusionist does. And even if you are going in for a procedure, still no-one is likely to explain the role of the perfusionist. Yet like the drummer in a band, they may not be the most high-profile member of the team, but they are absolutely critical to achieving a successful performance.

But no matter how important they may be to the process, perfusionists rarely get the recognition which the surgeons and nursing staff receive. Jenny Gavin, one of the perfusionists I am here to meet, mentioned that in more than twenty years neither she nor the perfusion department had ever received a thank you card from a patient. The next time I go in I will take a card and a box of chocolates to show my appreciation.

Jenny has now been a perfusionist at Blackpool for more than twenty-three years. She actually started her career as an intensive care nurse in Manchester but soon realised that nursing was not for her. Why was that, I asked? "I hated taking orders!" Hearing this, raucous laughter broke out from her colleagues. After nine years on the wards, she was given the opportunity to do a perfusionist job. She didn't know too much about it but decided to give it a try.

I learn how the training has changed so much over the years and that Jenny's journey into the role was much easier than it is for Ollie, who I am also here to meet. Ollie is the newest member of the team, having been with the department for just one year, and is still undergoing his training. To qualify these days, you have to do an MSc and perform 150 supervised cases coupled with significant external observation and testing.

Andy explains that Ollie's application stood out to him. It was not a normal degree or nursing pathway. It stood out because Ollie had come from a similar background to Andy. They both left school and went into painting and decorating before realising they wanted to do something different. It would be fair to say that being a perfusionist wasn't Ollie's first choice. He originally wanted to get into diagnostics but unfortunately did not get offered the post, so he looked into other options. Even though Ollie was looking for a career in cardiac care, he admits that he too was unfamiliar with what a perfusionist was and what they did. He only heard about it by seeing a couple of adverts. Though Ollie now feels he has found his vocation in life and finds his work exciting. He tells me that no two days are ever the same, that he never knows quite what to expect.

The third member of Andy's team I am here to meet is Marco. Marco studied biochemistry and had originally planned a career in academia. Before undertaking his PhD, Marco realised academia wasn't for him and opted for a change of direction. Like Ollie and Andy, Marco went through a period in limbo. He spent some time in compulsory military service in his native Greece. Afterwards, he spent time working as a toy salesman before finding his way into a private hospital which practised cardiac surgery. That was his introduction to perfusion. Marco went on to train at the biggest cardiac centre in the UK, the world-renowned Papworth Hospital, before making his way to Blackpool. It became apparent to me that, notwithstanding the necessity of advanced training, there are still many different roads to becoming a perfusionist.

After the meeting concluded, Andy asked me to accompany him on a little walk. As we headed down the corridor, he began to tell me of an incident which took place a week earlier. An eighteen-year-old Blackpool girl had been swept out in the freezing January sea. By the time the coast guard got to her, she had been adrift for at least half an hour.

The coast guard transferred her to an ambulance who immediately took her to A&E at Blackpool Victoria. Her body temperature on arrival was mid-20 degrees Celcius. To put that in perspective, the normal body temperature is 37c. Andy explains that once the heart's temperature drops down into the twenties, it tends to become arrhythmic and will eventually stop. This had unfortunately happened to this young lady.

The A&E team tried to work their magic with CPR and shock treatment but unfortunately, the girl did not respond. They were all for pronouncing her dead when someone mentioned that the cardiac team might have an answer. The patient was rushed up to the cardiac centre where a perfusionist was waiting to warm her blood using the bypass machine. By that point, it had been more than two hours since she had fallen into the sea. As the blood passed through the pump and began to warm up, miraculously the heart started beating again.

We arrived at CICU and Andy subtly pointed the patient out to me. I asked Andy if she was likely to suffer any long-term health problems. At this point, it would seem that she was making an astonishing recovery. The Lancashire Cardiac Centre deserve immense praise for achieving such a staggering outcome from what most people, even medical professionals, would have declared a lost cause.

Hearing this made me wonder whether anything like this had ever happened before. It turns out in February 2015, a twenty-five-year-old Pennsylvania man named Justin Smith was walking home in below-freezing temperatures. He had been having a few drinks with friends and at some point, along the way home, Justin blacked out. He wasn't found until the next morning when his father, Don Smith, saw his son lying by the road. According to the Lehigh Valley Health Network, the college student was in the snow for hours as the temperature plunged to four degrees below zero. Justin had no pulse and was presumed dead. His father said, "His face was blue, his body lifeless. I checked for a pulse, I checked for a heartbeat, there was nothing."

When Don Smith called paramedics, they did not give up on him. They commenced CPR with chest compressions but to no avail. Dr Gerald Coleman, an emergency physician at Lehigh Valley Hospital, had Smith rushed to the hospital for care. "You're not dead until you're warm and dead," Coleman said, referring to a phenomenon in which people who are kept at cold temperatures can be revived despite a lack of vital signs.

When Smith was brought into the emergency room, Coleman couldn't even get an accurate body temperature reading because Smith was so cold.

Undeterred, he transferred Smith via helicopter to a hospital where he could be hooked up to a machine called an ECMO (extracorporeal membrane oxygenation) similar to a bypass pump and also operated by a perfusionist. They used the ECMO machine to warm the patient's blood.

Dr James Wu, a cardiothoracic surgeon at Leigh Valley Hospital, thought it was still a long shot that Smith could survive. Yet ninety minutes after the machine was turned on, the young man's heart started to beat on its own.

It's not unheard of for film directors to establish working relationships with the same actors. Think of Francis Ford Copolla and Marlon Brando. Or Martin Scorsese and Robert De Niro. Similarly, members of the theatre team like to work with familiar colleagues where possible, the same surgeons, anaesthetists, perfusionists, and nursing staff. They do this because they develop a mutual understanding and professional bond. I met one scrub nurse, Neil, who had a book which contained all the preferences and personal quirks of each surgeon.

However, like a rock band or a cast of actors in a long-running production, new people can introduce a fresh perspective or innovation which might increase performance. I believe I met such a person on the corridor of the cardiac theatres. A friend of mine, Gary, was about to have heart surgery. I contacted him and we met up. He told me his surgeon was Mr Laskawski, one of the 'new kids on the block' at Blackpool. I had heard Mr Laskawski was doing some pretty amazing minimal invasive heart surgery. He had recently featured in an article in the Daily Mail along with another cardiothoracic surgeon, also at Blackpool, Mr Zacharias. They had worked together on the first keyhole repair of hypertrophic cardiomyopathy (thickening of the heart's septum) in the UK.

Consultant Cardiac Surgeon Mr Laskawski – His story
A consultant surgeon of Polish descent, Greg Laskawski became a member of the team at Blackpool following training in Poland and a period in Aberdeen. He is one of the younger generation of consultants and very keen on pushing himself outside of his comfort zone. It became clear when I had the chance to interview him that Greg Laskawski enjoys working at the frontier. He reminds me very much of the Wright Brothers, wanting to prove that the impossible might just be possible. Minimally invasive heart surgery requires a whole new skill set along with use of specialist methods and cutting-edge technology.

For the patient, the chief benefits of minimally invasive surgery are in the recovery period. Recovery is believed to be much quicker as you don't have your chest opened up and sewn back together. All you have is a small 6cm incision in the side of your chest wall just big enough to get the instruments through. But a shortening of recovery times and better overall outcomes is not a simple matter of deploying fancy tools. Success depends on surgeons like Mr Laskawski and his colleague Mr Zacharias having the passion to innovate.

Andrew Duncan had told me that back in the early days of cardiac surgery, virtually every heart operation was innovative. There were very few protocols or recognised procedures and in those early days, surgeons weren't under the same scrutiny. Failure was virtually an everyday occurrence and accepted as par for the territory. The surgery itself was also the primary focus back then whereas nowadays, a greater deal of emphasis is laid on the periods before and after the surgery. Greg explained how innovative rehabilitation techniques such as the Enhanced Recovery After Surgery programme (ERAS) are now critical to the entire process.

Listening to Mr Laskawski's passion for trying new things made me think of NASA's Apollo Moon programme. Much of the practical element was untried although all the research and the calculations suggested it should work. But what if it didn't? What if they had overlooked something? The outcome could be catastrophic. This was evidenced with Apollo 1 when they lost three astronauts in a fire during a simulation exercise just days before lift-off.

When you are dealing with human life, the stakes don't get any higher.

I was curious to learn about Greg's motivation to become a heart surgeon. He told me that when he was in medical school students would find themselves in one of two camps. Those who wanted to do something with their hands such as surgery and those who wanted to do research, medicine, or become GP's. Finding he inclined toward cardiac surgery, Mr Laskawski soon realised that this was probably the most demanding of all the medical specialities. He knew that it would be a lifetime commitment.

To be successful, he would need an incredible work ethic, passion, and the ability to cope with enormous amounts of stress. This would not be a 9-to-5 job. Exceptionally long days, weekends, and evenings were guaranteed but most significantly, he would have the incredible responsibility of people's lives literally in his hands. Listening to him reminded me yet again that cardiac surgeons are a very unique and special strain of human beings.

All of the surgeons I have had the privilege to interview all say that to get to where they are, they had to achieve much higher qualifications and experience than those required by the formal training programme. Mr Laskawski is no exception He gives me a fascinating insight into how he would go into the A&E department of his local hospital in Gdansk to see surgeons performing emergency surgery. He would spend every free hour he had watching and learning techniques and marvelling how cool-headed these surgeons were in such a highly charged environment.

I asked about the differences, if any, between working in the UK and working back home in Poland. Interestingly enough, in Poland, the surgeon makes the decision on what procedure the patient will undertake based on the information at hand. Yet in the UK, the patient is presented with all the options available to them and the surgeon always allows the patient the final call in which route they wish to take. Greg once had an 85-year-old patient who required valve replacement surgery. This man opted for a mechanical valve rather than a tissue valve which would have been the choice for a man of his mature years. When asked why, the patient said his mother lived until she was 105, as did many of his family, so he wanted a valve that would last. He didn't want to be coming back in ten years' time for a replacement.

I had always been curious about the relationships between surgeons and patients. Now, my own experience with cardiac surgery was unique. I came back *to meet my consultant again and ultimately ended up being part of the furniture, whilst writing this book.*

But most patients see their surgeons for only a short time. I asked Mr Laskawski if he could remember the names of patients that he operated on two weeks ago. His answer was very honest. He said on average, he does procedures 2-3 days a week with at least two procedures each day. If it's a straightforward procedure with no complications, then he probably can't recall them by name. However, if they experienced complications or there was something unique about the case, then he does tend to remember them. This is understandable when you stop to consider it. The department does around 1,300 surgical procedures each year, split between a small team of surgeons. Some surgeons at Blackpool have thousands of procedures under their belts.

Now you may think surgeons don't have to be physically fit but remember they have to concentrate for many hours. Surgeons can be rooted to the same spot for several hours at a time, their feet stuck in the same position for hour after hour. Although they don't move far, the effort required to sustain that level of concentration is physically draining. This is to say, nothing of the muscle memory required to pull off such intricate manoeuvres in such confined space again and again. During my numerous visits to theatre, I would gaze in astonishment at the dexterity of the surgeon and the complex manoeuvres they performed with their hands. Though notwithstanding the obvious physical demands, mentally surgeons have to be incredibly strong too. Many times, throughout the course of their careers, surgeons will be presented with a crisis, and they will be the person everybody looks to resolve it.

In my corporate training days, we used to do an exercise called "The Plank". We would put a wooden plank on the ground and ask team members to walk across it. Nobody hesitated and would even question the reason for doing such a menial task. That was until we suspended the plank twenty foot in the air. We gave them the same simple challenge: just walk across it. It was the same plank and the same task just twenty feet in the air. Suddenly it became a major psychological challenge. The confidence they had when it was on the floor evaporated.

Earlier in this chapter, I mentioned professional footballers who could perform Monday to Friday but on the big day when rehearsal becomes the real thing, they did not have the mental strength to cope. The plank is a great example of how mental strength can evaporate when the heat is on. I have met some incredibly determined people on this journey. People who would look at the plank twenty feet in the air and just go for it. Healthcare professionals who have taken on the ultimate challenge and have made great sacrifices to get to where they are.

How lucky are we to know these people are there when we need help?

When you are in theatre, most of the time, there is a lot of banter and as just mentioned, music playing. However, without the surgeon so much as uttering a word, all that would stop when they came to a demanding part of the procedure. Such is the subtlety of communication within the theatre team. The surgeon is like the conductor of an orchestra. Following a subtle glance or shift in posture, akin to the slightest flick of the conductor's baton, the players know what to do.

One thing fascinated me. Did the heart rate of the surgeons themselves, in deep concentration at critical moments of the procedure, rise? Cardiac surgery is incredibly stressful, even though the surgeons often give off an aura of calm and confidence. There's a saying that cardiac surgery can be 'awfully simple or simply awful.'

I wondered if this old man had the cojones to pose to a world-class heart surgeon that they should wear a Holter heart monitor (a device used to monitor the heart rate of patients) in theatre as an experiment? After all, what would the results say about the surgeon? How would colleagues interpret the results? Surgeons can be a very competitive group and any perceived weakness might be exploited! How would it be interpreted if the heart rate went sky high? What if it never fluctuated? As a consultant surgeon, could becoming involved with such a hare-brained idea put your reputation on the line?

The day came when I had planned to meet with Mr Walker and his registrar Ms Toolan. We were going to talk about being a trainee and the challenges trainees face, especially as a female. As

I have an hour's journey to get to the hospital, I found myself thinking "today's the day to float the heart monitor idea." But how? I arrived at the hospital via the main entrance. A shimmer of pensiveness took over.

By now, I had visited the hospital many times over what seemed like a very short period. First as a patient, now as a writer. I passed the volunteers, easily identifiable in their orange shirts, and said hello. Costa was heaving, as normal and it was just a little past eight in the morning.

As I climbed the flights of stairs up to the second floor where the theatres and offices were located, I considered my options for suggesting the heart monitor experiment and wondered what the worst outcome could be. Perhaps I could be thrown out onto the street, never to be invited back again! I began to consider the content I had acquired so far. If I ended up face down chewing Tarmac, could I finish the book from here? I believed I could. So, I came up with what I thought was a sure-fire solution, as long as I didn't bottle it at the last minute.

As always, I was greeted warmly by Mr Walker and Ms Toolan. We spent the first few minutes talking about what had happened since my last visit. The conversation was flowing easily and at one point, we were all laughing. This, I thought, was the moment to drop the question. "Wouldn't it be fascinating to put heart monitors on you to see how your hearts perform when you are undertaking a procedure?" I closed my eyes and waited for a big hand to grab me and escort me to the roadside, but the response was not what I was expecting. Mr Walker exclaimed, "what a great idea!" I breathed a sigh of relief and excitement began to fill the air.

For the next ten minutes, we discussed the idea and agreed that we should do it as soon as we could get the monitors from the Cardiac Investigations Unit. It was agreed that Jordan, Mr Walker's secretary, would arrange to get the monitors and he would let me know when they would be available.

The day after my meeting was Friday. I receive an email from Jordan saying that he had managed to get the monitors for Tuesday. "Which Tuesday?" I replied. "Next Tuesday," came his response, bouncing back. "Blimey," I thought, normally you have to wait weeks.

Tuesday came and I arrived at the hospital around eight-thirty in the morning. I put on my theatre scrubs ready to watch Mr Walker and Ms Toolan perform miracles in the operating theatre. Mr Walker and Ms Toolan had been wired up with the monitors since seven o'clock, so we had already had a good hour and a half plus of monitoring. It was agreed that Ms Toolan, who was at this time, nearing the completion of her final exam, could start the procedure with Mr Walker nearby, if required.

The two procedures were fairly standard, and the day passed without any major alarms, or did they? The heart monitors were to be left on until seven o'clock the following morning. A member of the theatre team said with a smile on their face, "Be careful what you get up to tonight." I had no idea what they were suggesting.

A day later and I received an email that the results were available with the question, "When can you come in?" Keen to know the outcome, I agreed to be there the following morning.

In his own words, here is Tony Walker's interpretation of the data:

OK. It's official.

Two or three times per day, two or three days per week, I touch someone's heart. Not metaphorically speaking. I mean, I actually touch someone's heart. As a cardiac surgeon, that's par for the course.

I touch it. I stop it. Hopefully, mend it. Usually, though sometimes with help, I start it going again.

Despite that, it's official. I'm boring.

During the twenty-four hours, I was being monitored, a lot happened. Although not, apparently, with my own cardiac activity.

Sawing through the breast-bone of my patient, 68 beats per minute; placing a large tube in the biggest artery in the body (the aorta), 68 beats per minute; stitching 2-3-millimetre tubes together, 68 beats per minute; stopping the heart, 68 beats per minute; replacing a damaged heart valve, 67 beats per minute; stopping the bypass machine and making sure the patient's heart is working well enough to keep them alive, 65 beats per minute.

Over 86,000 beats in twenty-four hours and not once did it get over 100 beats per minute. In fact, most of the time, it hovered around 60 beats per minute.

During the same period, my registrar was monitored in exactly the same way. She left me way behind; over 103,000 beats during the twenty-four hours and she had tachycardia (a heart rate over 100 beats per minute) for 12% of the day. In comparison, I'd spent over a quarter of my day with bradycardia (a slow heart rate of fewer than 60 beats per minute).

The simple explanation is not that I was asleep in my office (or strolling around the golf course, as seems to be the public's image of the consultant surgeon), whilst she did the day's work. We worked together. We shared the tasks and, hopefully, I taught her how to do aspects of the surgery. In fact, for one case she did it all.

I watched. I resisted the urge to interfere. I let her begin to establish her own approach and techniques, hopefully, in a safe and supported way. It was hard.

I was desperate to comment. To guide; to assist; to join in; to do it my tried and tested way. But, physiologically, at least as far as my own heart was concerned, it was a doddle: 65 beats per minute.

Clearly, I'm not boring.

My years of training and consultant practice have given my brain experience and I've built mental models, road maps to subconsciously follow; my hands and forearms have muscle memory for the different techniques and procedures they perform. So, it would seem my heart and physiology have memory too, providing a calm, constant environment in which everything else I do in theatre can work smoothly.

This experience cannot be hurried or implanted; its gained. Could physiological stability such as this be an accurate marker of skill and expertise? Perhaps a twenty-four-hour monitor such as this should become an integral part of the consultant surgeon interview? Or perhaps it's just a one-off and next week I'll be palpitating, sweating, and shaking with the rest of them!

As with everything I do in my work, this one simple challenge has prompted more questions, thoughts, and uncertainties that need to be explored; the joy and excitement of cardiac surgery.

One period Mr Walker did leave out was they both had a spike around nine o'clock in the evening. When I asked as to why, Tony said it was at a time when he was waiting for a colleague to arrive to help with one of his patients who had become distressed. For Caroline, it was when she couldn't get the microwave working to warm up her supper. It seems the coolness demonstrated by a cardiac surgeon under the most intense pressure can be undone by a faulty microwave and the lateness of a colleague! Maybe this simple little experiment has uncovered some really useful scientific data?

Ms Toolan finished her final exam and left the department soon after we conducted this experiment. Her training in Blackpool was at its conclusion and she was heading back to Liverpool, but not before I had a chance to interview her.

Reader Question

Think about the challenges you have taken on in your life.

What would you do differently if you had the chance to experience them again in order to achieve a better end result?

Chapter 6

The Ward Round

**"Give every day the chance to become the
most beautiful day of your life."**

At this point in my journey, I have spent a lot of
time with consultants and theatre staff. What I need
is to increase my understanding of how a cardiac
ward operates. I have arranged to spend a night
shift on CICU to get a feel for working through the
night and to see how staff cope with patients at
their most vulnerable. The only other time I had
been in CICU was as a patient and those few days
were a bit of a blur.

I arrive to find that registrar Ms Hardman,
who I have already met, was on call. Any
emergencies or surgical input through the night
will be her responsibility. I had previously watched
her do several surgical procedures and had gained
immense respect for her abilities. She is one of the
new generation, out to make their mark. We should
be in safe hands tonight.

We meet in the coffee room and I ask what a
night on call is typically like. Apparently, it varies
a lot. Some nights, you can get some hours rest and
others can be constant work. We finish our coffees
and head over to CICU. All is eerily quiet. I have
never been in the hospital at night before and so the
silence caught me off guard. As we do a walk
around, stopping at each patient, Ms Hardman
looks at the chart at the end of each bed. Many
cardiac centres have gone digital with this info but

Blackpool still prefers the written word on a large chart. Ms Hardman has a few words with each nurse before moving on.

As we continue to check in on the patients, I see people looking just how I would have looked during my stay on CICU. There are people on ventilation, others with drains or drips in situ. I recall all the tubes and monitoring equipment I was hooked up to. It's hard, being in a place like this, not to feel a bizarre sense of nostalgia. Waking up in here, and everything that followed, set me on the path I'm now walking. I wonder where life will take these patients once they leave here?

Once we finish the ward round, Ms Hardman leaves me in the company of sister Debbie who is busy catching up with lots of reports and other admin. Debbie has been a nurse for twenty-five years and seems to love her job. I ask her why she enjoys the critical care end of nursing? Her response is similar to others I have interviewed. Ultimately, she takes pride in quality care and helping very poorly people get better. It must give great satisfaction to see someone leave the ward in better health.

I take a seat next to Debbie on the front desk. Before us, are several screens displaying the vital signs of people in the beds all around us. Gazing at these screens, I am reminded of the gravity of this line of work. As Debbie continues with her admin work, I glance at the clock. It says the time is now 3:00 am. So far, the night has been very quiet, which of course is exactly what you want it to be. Still, I can feel the tension all around. Perhaps it's my inexperience in this kind of environment but just being around people in critical dependency is enough to set my nerves on edge as I preempt an alarm to go off. Each bleep from the monitors snatches my attention and yet the nurses seem calm, totally at home in this unique environment.

I look at the clock again, it is now nearly 5:am. Suddenly, the sun starts to stream through the windows. As this summer's day dawns, a whole new set of challenges face the unit as downstairs more new patients will be arriving for their procedures. I say my goodbyes to Debbie and the staff and head out into the pale morning light.

As I'm driving home, I begin to dwell on those patients I had just spent the night with. Each one of them a mother, brother, best friend. I'm filled with wistful sentiments, a reverence for the fragility of life. Heart disease does not discriminate as celebrities like Barry Manilow, Bill Clinton and Arnold Schwarzenegger might well testify. It affects old and young. Rich and poor. As my wife Helen and I can attest, you never really know what's around the corner.

On the drive home and for whatever reason, a specific Queen song popped into my head. The song, *"These are the Days of our Lives"* was one of the last songs Freddie wrote. The first verse went like this:

> *Sometimes I get to feelin'*
> *I was back in the old days, long ago*
> *When we were kids, when we were young*
> *Things seemed so perfect, you know?*
> *The days were endless, we were crazy, we were young*
> *The sun was always shinin', we just lived for fun*

When we're young we lack the furrows of worry and responsibility which come with maturity. Yet when sickness and old age descends it brings things into focus. What do we want to live for? Why are we here? Even one night on the unit is enough to rouse my heart. What must it be like for those nurses whose daily lives are spent working with patients whose lives are about to be changed forever?

A few days pass and I am on my way to observe a shift on Ward 37. This is the cardiology ward where patients who can be managed medically will be cared for. It is filled with patients admitted with heart attacks, arrhythmias, and other conditions which don't yet require the attention of a cardiac surgeon. Some patients are here to have a pacemaker fitted or battery changed. There are even some non-cardiac patients dotted around owing to bed shortages elsewhere in the hospital.

It's another early start today as I need to be on the ward for 7:30am. This is when the shift changeover happens and the briefing session for the inbound shift takes place. When I arrive, I am greeted by Rachel the ward sister.

The new shift has arrived, and the team is waiting to receive the briefing from the outgoing shift. There are eleven people in the room. The briefing contains a full review of the night's activities and each patient's progress from the outgoing shift. It takes a little while to cover all thirty-three beds on the ward. Among the team taking over, I counted a ward manager, a ward sister (Rachel), four or five staff nurses, five healthcare assistants, one housekeeper, two ward clerks and a student nurse. Throughout the day, the ward plays host to other healthcare professionals such as physiotherapists, doctors, and other practitioners so the team can grow quite considerably over the course of the day. The meeting finishes and the team set out onto the ward.

Rachel takes me behind the reception. The desk is well-staffed and stacked with case notes, reports, and monitors displaying vital signs similar to those I had seen on CICU. Again, I am reminded of how serious this place is. Behind reception is a big white box with what looks like a large drainpipe protruding from it. I stare at it curiously as it begins to clatter and rumble. After a few moments, a large plastic tube shoots out from within. What is this contraption? Apparently, there is a labyrinth of hidden piping throughout the hospital which carries these plastic cylinders to their various destinations. I'm told it's the quickest way to get blood that needs analysing over to the pathology lab.

It's now 8:00am and breakfast time is upon us. A huge stainless-steel carriage is wheeled in and the health care assistants gather around to take the pre-selected breakfasts to the patients.

8:00am is also when Rachel performs some of the most vital daily checks of ward equipment. She takes me over to have a look at the resuscitation trolley. This contains defibrillators, an oxygen cylinder, and other equipment to assist with cardiac arrests. I ask how often it is used, Rachel tells me it can be used three times a week or it can sit there for months. Touch wood, I haven't witnessed anything frightening yet. But the potential is always lingering, and the staff clearly take preparation very seriously.

One of the roles Rachel finds challenging is delivering the bad news to patients when their procedures are delayed or cancelled. There is an elderly lady, Betty, who has been in for a day or two. She lives alone with no family nearby. She had a fall and came to the hospital in an ambulance via A&E. The lady has very low blood pressure which had led her to lose consciousness. Betty had thought she would be having a pacemaker fitted today but word had just come through that the procedure would have to be postponed. It was now down to Rachel to inform Betty what had happened.

I accompany Rachel to Betty's bedside where she is sitting in a chair gazing out of the window. Rachel enters the room with such a radiant smile it is difficult not to warm to her. She leans forward and quietly delivers Betty's disappointing news. Betty's countenance says it all. Her high-cheeked smile sinks in resignation. She is devastated. Rachel assures Betty that Dr Roberts will be on the ward shortly and will give her an update. I can't help but feel a pang of sadness as we leave Betty to digest the bad news.

Back out on the ward, the pace is growing. There is so much to do. Reception is continually busy with people coming and going. The two ward clerks, Julie and Jane, are doing battle with the telephones as family and friends call in to see how their loved ones have fared overnight. A number of nurses were busy conducting the medication rounds. At 9:00am the physiotherapists from the rehab team hit the ward and Rachel is whisked off to meet with them.

I join a healthcare assistant named Julie on her morning rounds. Julie is hard at work changing beds, replenishing water, and moving patients around so they don't get bed sores. She tells me managing bedsores take up a lot of her time.

Healthcare assistants are the glue that holds the ward together. The very nature of their work means they spend most of their time in patient contact. In fact, they can develop such a relationship with patients that doctors may ask a healthcare assistant to accompany them when giving bad news.

Another healthcare assistant, Adele, comes over to assist Julie. Adele is a spritely lady with a very distinctive walk. She has always been in the care business through care homes and has spent ten years on Ward 37. I quickly come to realise that Adele is a real character. I ask everyone I interview if they have any funny stories and most people struggle to recall them when put on the spot. But not Adele. She reeled them off like a stand-up comedian, launching into a tale of how she once asked a paraplegic gentleman to swing his legs over the bed. Luckily, the patient saw the funny side. Having barely paused for breath she tells me about the time when she put the incinerator out of action by putting the whole bedpan in rather than just the cardboard bit. On another occasion, she started a new job and sat in on the shift changeover for 30 minutes before realising she was on the wrong ward. I can understand how Adele has found her calling in health care. I've only been with her for ten minutes and she has brightened the room.

It's 11:00am and it's time for the consultant's ward round. Today the consultant on call is Dr Roberts who very kindly allows me to join him on his round. Dr Roberts has been at Blackpool for many years, long before the new cardiac centre was opened. He has many stories to tell about how the department has developed over the years. He told me about the role Labour MP Alan Milburn and Sir Roger Boyle played in making it happen. Throughout a decade long modernisation effort, the government made heart disease a priority bringing the national waiting time for a procedure down from eighteen months to just eighteen weeks.

As we move from one patient to the next, Dr Roberts shows everyone dignity and respect. He addresses most of the patients by their first names. Each is given the time they need and, if necessary, Dr Roberts would request further investigations or amendments to the medication before moving on. He never hurried anybody.

At the conclusion of the ward round, Rachel catches up with us and asks if I would like to go on the morning break with her. Another cup of tea sounds like just what I need at that moment, so I say a big thank you to Dr Roberts and follow Rachel into the coffee room. I want to know more about Rachel's life and how she got into this profession.

Ward Sister Rachel – Her story

Rachel was actually born in the Blackpool Victoria Hospital, the very hospital we are in. She has strong family ties to 'the Vic' as her Mum was also a nurse here and it was on Ward 11 that her mum and dad first met.

Rachel was a late starter, beginning her training when she was twenty-four. Before this, she did her A-Levels and spent some time working as a health care assistant. After some time, she applied for paramedic training and was awarded a place. This made Rachel realise she is a home bird at heart and didn't want to move away! So, Rachel ended up leaving healthcare altogether and started work as a receptionist at Ribby Hall, a local hotel.

One day Rachel turned up for work and sat down to a day like any other. She took phone calls, answered queries. She chatted with customers. Suddenly a young boy rushed in asking her to phone an ambulance. His grandfather was feeling very dizzy. Rachel went to see the man and realised he was having a cardiac arrest. Seeing this poor man suffering changed Rachel's view on what she wanted to do with her life. It seemed fate was conspiring to bring her back to the Vic.

Inspired, she applied to do her nurse training and had soon completed her first placement on Ward 37. This time, it was for real. She loved it so much she didn't want to move. Five years ago, she applied to become the Ward Sister. She was one of two applicants and got the job by half a point in the scoring system. But promotion was a big step for Rachel. She didn't realise that the blue uniform was like a magnet for anyone who had a question or needed advice. With fifty staff around, there are plenty of people wanting questions answered or advice!

In the last few years, Rachel has had a baby girl and now lives in Chorley, Lancashire. Chorley has its own large hospital, but Rachel prefers to work at the Vic as it feels like a second home to her. Rachel has made many friends on the ward, both colleagues and patients. Her best friends are also her work colleagues. Being here, listening to the camaraderie between the staff, it feels like a real community. There's just something of a buzz about the place. I get the feeling that life on the ward can be quite colourful, so I probe for some amusing tales. Rachel ponders for a second before recalling having a jacket potato thrown at her head by an elderly woman. Luckily Rachel's reflexes were too sharp.

Now, with thirty-three patients on the ward, it's difficult to keep track of them all. They have a system where a patient leaving the ward for a walk or going to the shop must sign a register, so the staff know where they have gone. One day, an older gentleman signed the book and said he was just popping off to the shop. Some considerable time later, the man returned dressed in his outdoor clothes. Bemused, Rachel asked where he'd been. He told her he had been on the bus into town to get his trousers changed! Security is a lot tighter nowadays.

Though it's not all laughter, life on the ward can be humbling and sad. Sometimes patients can stay for many weeks or months. It's natural for people to grow fond of one another, essentially living together for such long periods, meeting their friends and relatives. Losing a patient, you've got to know can be very upsetting. Rachel told me of a story about one man sitting in his chair waiting for his wife to come and see him. Suddenly, alarms began blaring. Cardiac arrest staff rushed to assist but sadly he passed away just as his wife arrived. I'm stunned. It's difficult to imagine how everybody must have felt. Life as a sister on a cardiac ward must be

extremely   demanding   but   hopefully,   extremely
rewarding

Back to the ward. I am busy scribbling notes next to the reception desk when a man walked in with a supermarket bag full of chocolates and biscuits. He asks if a certain staff member is in work today. Unfortunately, it's her day off. One of the nurses on duty recognises him and rushes over for a hug. The man was in for several weeks under observation. He was so impressed with the care he received he just wanted to show his gratitude. After he had left, I asked Rachel if many people come back to say thanks like this. By way of response, Rachel took me to a wall that was literally covered with hundreds of thank you cards.

The mad rush of the morning has now subsided, so Rachel takes me to meet Julia the practice development manager. Luckily, she has a moment for a quick chat and so we find a quiet office to sit down to chat.

Practice Development Manager Julia - Her story
Julia plays an educational role in the cardiac nursing team and is responsible for the training requirements of each of the 120 nurses on the wards. She is responsible for their professional journey and making sure they are equipped with the right skill set.

Julia was born and bred in Lytham St Annes, just a few miles down the road from the hospital and went to university in Hull to do her nurse training. From there, she followed her husband to Birmingham and worked on the cardiac wards of Queen Elizabeth Hospital. Julia and her husband would eventually return to the Fylde coast to start a family. Julia joined the cardiac team at Blackpool Victoria and became ward manager before applying for the post of practice development manager. Julia's days can be very varied. Some days are classroom-based, others she spends responding to the many emails she receives. Julia is very passionate about what she does, telling me that she can think about her day long into the night.

Julia feels a bit like a "mother hen" in her role. She had organised a training session a few weeks earlier which was supposed to start at 9:00am but then nurses are not used to starting at nine, so people were coming in at different times. It was a larger than normal group and some of the formats had been changed. After thirty minutes, someone burst out laughing and said "Julia, it's like you're trying to herd frogs." She tells me that the hardest part of the job is asking nurses to get involved in sessions when they are already totally committed and focused on patient care.

As a release from work and to get some work-life balance, Julia loves her garden and spends many hours in it.

After yet another fascinating day, I find myself heading home again. Since starting this journey, the drive home gives me the time to reflect on life and the paths we take and the people I've met. People like Rachel, Marko, and Ollie. People like Dr Chalil and Mr Bose who have committed their lives to the care of others.

I remember being younger, sitting cross-legged in front of the TV watching *Blue Peter*. Valerie Singleton was interviewing an airline pilot who had been responsible for flying some extremely rare Egyptian artefacts over to the UK. Valerie asked him if that was the most valuable cargo he had ever flown. The pilot quickly responded, "nothing is more valuable than 200 passengers putting their lives in your hands." Looking very embarrassed Ms Singleton replied, "what a great answer." Egyptian artefacts, no matter how valuable, cannot come close to the value of human life.

Reader Question

Consider where you are in your life.

How could you improve just one area to make life better?

Chapter 7

Second Life and a New Buddy

'There are only two days in the year where life is not possible, yesterday and tomorrow.

Today is the day to maximise your life'

So, the hard bit is behind you. The months if not years of suffering have finally concluded in the cardiac theatre, where for those few hours, you have had zero knowledge of what has been happening to you. Which is probably a good thing, although dedicated professionals have been doing some amazing things to your heart.

But now, it's time to bring you back to the real world. You have just woken up in CICU, where my first thought was, 'Wow I made it.' I believe most patients have that eureka moment when they open their eyes for the first-time post-procedure.

Even though you're awake, your body is still full of drugs, you are drifting in and out of consciousness you really have no idea what is going on just an overwhelming feeling of relief.

I strongly believe that to aid recovery and start your 'Second Life' positively, you need to set targets. For some patients I spoke to, this was a date for when they wanted to return to the golf course, for others it was a little less ambitious such as just being able to push a trolley around a supermarket. Everyone's target will be different. The key point is to have one.

The early stages of recovery are all about getting you mobile. Physiotherapists will come in and get you out of bed and moving as soon as they feel you are ready. The stay in CICU and on the cardiac wards are based on how quickly you get to the point of being mobile. There is a big dilemma at this point, as the system needs your bed for the next tranche of patients but obviously, no-one wants you to leave before you feel ready and able to cope back home.

The CICU team at the Lancashire Cardiac Centre realised the trauma of being in CICU for patients and their families so they decided to produce a video called 'A Patients Journey'. It was produced so patients and families could watch prior to the procedure to help demystify the journey and help them understand the process and the monitoring equipment the patient would be hooked up to in CICU, with the intention to reduce the shock when seeing it for the first time.

CICU has twenty critical care beds with a hundred staff over the shift patterns to nurture you back to health. I have been privileged to have spent a night shift on the unit and was incredibly impressed with the passion and dedication of the team who work in critical health care.

The ratio of nurses to patients depends on the level of care required by the patient. If the patient requires ventilation, help with breathing, they will have their own dedicated nurse 24/7. If the patient is what is called 'high dependency', then the ratio is 2:1. Either way, the care is world-class and a tribute to the team who look after us.

Because the care is so individual, so personal, the nursing staff do get to know their patients and families quite intimately. I remember an hour-long conversation with Daniel, one of the nurses who looked after me and thinking, shouldn't he be somewhere else? Its conversations like these where the nurses can get a good insight and evaluate any patient or family issues with the resource to help direct them to the best possible solution available.

I have done the patient journey, but I was fascinated to know what the 'Second Life' journey was like from a family members perspective. So, I met Sue, whose husband David, had had heart surgery.

Heart disease patient spouse Sue - Her story
Sue is the wife of David, a couple who contacted me via a newspaper article written about me and my passion to develop a professional support group. I wanted to get David's journey through the eyes of a family member to see how their journey differs from the patients.

Sue agreed to meet me at Wilf's, a café where we can sit outside in the sunshine.

Sue has been married to David for more than forty years. Most marriages after forty years have probably lost a bit of 'Je Ne Sais Quoi' but not David and Sue; they openly admit that they are as close today as they were forty years ago.

To fast forward a little bit, David had felt unwell, so with Sue by his side, he undertook a number of visits to his GP followed by cardiologists who came to the conclusion David had a heart murmur. He was told it wasn't serious, so to carry on as normal.

On one of the rare days when David and Sue were not together, David decided to walk up a local fell on his own. The start of the walk is extremely steep, and David found he needed to stop on a number of occasions. On reaching a plateau, David remembers sitting on a rock but then passing out. Although David didn't know it at the time, a couple on the same walk had called for an ambulance.

The next thing David remembers is being in the A&E dept at Barrow hospital.

His next destination, after more consultations, was the Lancashire Cardiac Centre at Blackpool where he met consultant surgeon, Mr Andrew Duncan. Sue was keen to know what the process was. She was reassured by nurses that Mr Duncan was the senior surgeon and David was in the best place with the best consultant.

An angiogram, which all patients undertaking heart surgery must have, was arranged. It was after this that Sue noticed David was a bit 'wobbly'. As time progressed, Sue also noticed David was getting worse. He was getting breathless, feeling weaker and on occasions, felt the need to sit up in bed.

Finally, David got the date for his procedure and they prepared for the hour-long journey to Blackpool. I asked Sue if she could remember what they talked about on the way down. All she could remember is talking about other people's bad driving. I wondered if this was a deflection from the reality they were heading towards.

I ask Sue what she was thinking about when she knew David was having his procedure, her response was' no news is good news', based on the fact she would have received a call should anything untoward have happened.

Sue tells me she tried to keep to her daily routine as normal as possible all but for a couple of hours out, to drive down to see David. It was on a return journey when Sue remembers her heart started to pound. She got home and took her own blood pressure to find it was sky-high. A trip to the doctors endorsed that it was anxiety based on her concern for David. This became true as her anxiety passed once David was home.

Once home, Sue explains that David seemed very angry and frustrated, I personally can understand this because all the things you took for granted before the procedure now seem so difficult to achieve. Sue says she felt she was walking on eggshells, nervous about saying or doing the wrong thing.

I ask Sue if it would have been advantageous to have a third-party organisation or someone who had gone through the same situation to bounce the situation off? Her response was it could have been very helpful because she did feel she wanted to share her feelings with someone.

It was fascinating that when David arrived home, they didn't discuss how he was feeling, Sue continues, I guess David didn't want to worry her and she didn't want to nag him.

On their post-operative meeting with Mr Duncan, she was asked what he was like when he got home, Sue replied, "He was a miserable git," but then felt guilty because she realised, he had gone through a pretty traumatic journey, but she admits she felt she needed a bit of attention herself.

For six months, David made steady progress before slipping into Atrial Fibrillation needing a cardioversion *to put his heart back into rhythm, followed by a catheter ablation.*

I ask Sue what her lowest emotional point was during the journey; she was quite adamant that it was when he came home and was so un-communitive.

I wanted to know if Sue was to take on the journey again, what would she like to see in place and what would she do differently? Her response was fascinating. She felt that partners and family members should be formally told what to expect from the patient when they get home both physically and mentally. "If you have some knowledge of what might happen, then you can be prepared for it, otherwise it's a journey into the unknown".

So, my final question was if the procedure increased her quality of life? Sue's reply was that it had given them back the life they had before the problem. With that and the fact that our cups had been collected a long time ago, made us realise we may have overstayed our welcome at the café.

For the first few days after returning home from my operation, I was questioning if all the strange feelings both physical and mental were normal. The first chance to ask someone was when the district nurse visited a week after you arrive home.

Everyone's journey is unique and that includes the speed of recovery. If I am at one end of the recovery spectrum being of more mature age, today I am going to meet a young man at the other end.

I am taking a trip to Colne in Lancashire to meet Marc, a thirty-five-year-old triathlete who found out he had a congenital heart condition and needed a valve replacement. I was particularly interested to interview him because he is one of the seven hundred fit young people each year who find they need a heart procedure.

I wanted to find out if there was any difference in how a young fit athlete would recover both mentally and physically from such traumatic surgery to that of a more mature patient.

I fall off the end of the M65 and take a few right and lefts before arriving at number thirty-one, Marc is sat outside, making the most of the early evening sun. He looks every bit the pro athlete. He has the stereotype sporting physic, very muscular and his face looks as though it's been chiselled out of granite. He invites me in, and we engage in idle chat before we start the interview.

Patient Marc - His story

Marc was born in Burnley, educated in Colne. During his school days, he was well into sport representing school and county in a number of sports. His main passion was football and at twelve years old, he was 'scouted' by Burnley FC.

The next bit of Marc's story will fly in the face of what most youngsters would have done. At the age when Burnley wanted to sign him professionally, he chose to follow an academic route. Marc is a sharp cookie. He was not blinded by the image of being a professional footballer but looking at the long-term game of what he wanted to do in life.

The academic journey took him to Loughborough University where he got a 1st class honours degree in

Business Economics. When you meet Marc, you can see he has a steely determination to succeed in whatever he does.

After a brief encounter with the Paras which a prolapsed disc put paid to, Marc joined the family business. Now with a stable working environment, Marc decided to get fit and was introduced to the incredibly challenging sport of triathlons.

Right from the outset, Marc was getting placed and realised he could probably make it to the top of the rankings. By 2017, Marc was performing at the highest level and getting placed. But then, all that changed. Over a number of competitions, Marc realised he was starting to get breathless but put it down to just starting to fast. From horizontal to vertical in the transition from swim to the bike, he was getting palpitations. In training, he was having to stop, things were not looking good. His heart rate monitor told him his heart rate was exceeding 200bpm.

One night, sat at home watching the TV, Marc realised even in relaxed mode, his heart was not right. It was suffering Atrial Fibrillation; his heart was beating erratically. It was this situation that Marc realised he needed to get checked out and made an appointment with the doctors. From here, the normal run of tests was carried out including an echocardiogram and other scans which showed he had congenital bicuspid aortic valve regurgitation.

Marc met Mr Walker initially in Blackburn and then in Blackpool. After more tests, it was decided he needed valve surgery and an aortic wrap around due to dilation of the artery.

There are two different types of valve available, a mechanical one and a tissue version. This was a major decision for Marc, as the mechanical one meant he would need to be on blood-thinning medication for the rest of his life. Doing the physical job he does and the nature of triathlons, there would always be a worry of injury and bleeding. So, Marc decided on the tissue valve, even though he may need another operation further down the line.

Marc being the person he is, started to do the research on tissue valves and came across one called the Edwards Resilia Valve which he felt was the best one for his lifestyle. Unfortunately, this was not an available option on the NHS as it was at least twice the cost of the normal tissue valves used within the Cardiac Centre. The benefits for this valve were that it had had considerable research done on it which other valves were lacking.

Again, with the determination of a highly competitive athlete, Marc and Mr Walker were able to convince the hospital this was a unique trial and acquired the necessary funding.

Marc said he didn't feel any anxiety as he had just accepted it as another challenge and faced it with the same determination he would adopt when approaching a triathlon.

Post-procedure, Marc did have a few minor blips which kept him in slightly longer than planned.

The speed of Marc's recovery was impressive. Being young and fit had a major, positive effect. With his strong competitive attitude, he told me he was running within a week of arriving home and had gone back to work just two days after leaving the hospital.

Ten weeks after surgery, every patient is offered a place on a rehab programme. Marc went to the first one, but the nurses said the programme would have zero benefits for him as he was way above the level the programme was aimed at.

When I asked patients where they want to be in five years' time, some say, 'hopefully still taking a breath' but Marc has a clear vision on where he wants to be. His target is to compete at the Iron Man World Championships in Hawaii.

Having spent a couple of hours in this incredible young man's company I don't believe there is any doubt he will achieve his ambition. Good luck Marc.

The area I feel left to the patient to manage is the emotional journey. Some people can cope with this element but some like myself struggle; so, how is this need identified and where do you go for support?

As already mentioned, the Cardiac department has two psychologists attached to it, to support patients who are emotionally suffering. However, before they can get involved an emotional issue would have to be identified, but who's responsibility is the emotional wellbeing of the patient. Surgeons are highly skilled in the art of 'fixing' the heart. They openly admit they are not psychologists.

Unlike a physical illness you can see, emotional wellbeing is difficult to assess as it all starts between the ears and no-one can see what's going on in there.

In my case, the anxiety-emotional-depression wheels came off some weeks after my return home. I suddenly started to wonder what had gone on in the six hours I have zero knowledge of on the day of my operation. What was different inside me?

Had the traumatic experience change me, not just physically but mentally? I don't believe I am the only one to have had what some psychologists call Critical Incident Stress Disorder.

It has to be said that the majority of heart patients tend to be mature and would benefit from having the support of family and friends on their return home. Recovery, when you're older, is considerably slower than Mark the triathlete mentioned earlier. Your body takes much longer to recover from the trauma of having your chest opened up, having the most important organ in your body repaired and having anaesthetic drugs pumped around you for a number of hours.

It is easy to find excuses not to do the exercises or walk as the physios have suggested. In my case it was January, freezing cold and icy.

It was during the weeks after arriving home that my mind became full of questions and 'what if's'. I really wanted and needed someone I could talk to, someone who had done the journey and was now much healthier and fitter for it. I needed an inspirational figure to help me through the traumatic journey that was starting to engulf me.

We all know how powerful the mind is, yet the NHS system does not seem to recognise how powerful it can be in helping or hindering a patient through a traumatic illness and recovery.

I have a vision of a concept I have called Buddy Beat. Buddy Beat would be a professional organisation run by a few paid staff and delivered by highly trained Buddy volunteers selected from patients who have undertaken the journey and are now living a much more productive and inspirational lifestyle.

A ten-week training programme would be undertaken and delivered by healthcare professionals. By the end of the programme, Buddies will be well versed in emotional intelligence, body language, psychology, counselling skills, and a knowledge of physiology and anatomy related to cardiac disease. They will also get the opportunity to experience a live theatre procedure.

Buddy Beat would raise the profile of the emotional, psychological and mentoring opportunities available to patients and families.

Buddy Beat is not a quick fix. It will require significant development and funding to create a professional strategy that includes recruitment, a ten-week training programme, Social media platforms, video production and a whole variety of interactive events.

To acquire the level of funding required, the project will need considerable scientific measurement to evaluate its success. Some of those measurement indicators will be accelerating recovery, patient emotional development, self-esteem, confidence and patients own feeling of wellbeing. We would propose doing a cohort group who do not have access to the Buddy system so we can evaluate the difference in recovery and overall feeling of positiveness and wellbeing throughout the journey.

This measurement tool would need to be independently developed ideally in conjunction with a university and scientifically evaluated. Many of the surgeon's support and want to be involved in the development of such a potential world-class programme.

We all believe having a university as a partner would give the programme credibility and be a fantastic academic model for students to evaluate and document all patients' wellbeing and recovery.

My view is that Buddy Beat is based loosely on the Samaritans concept, where it is more a listening friendship service. It is not an advice-giving service as the buddies won't be health care professionals. They do however have their own experience to draw on which will be priceless.

I have trained and been a Samaritan's counsellor for five years.

Families are almost as important as the patient in that they are on their own journey, watching their loved ones suffer. They suffer, not being able to help in a clinical way. Buddy Beat will offer families an arena where they can seek advice and information without upsetting their loved one, the patient.

I recently became a patient again in the Cardiac Centre and spent a night on Ward 38. This reinforced my belief that a buddy system is of paramount importance. I make that statement, not because the care was not good, it was as impeccable as it was the first time, but it did highlight my views that there is a whole side of healthcare and recovery which in my opinion creates a great opportunity.

When on the ward, the patient can have many, many hours of cerebral inactivity and stimulation. This is a time when negative thoughts can develop, and your emotional state can decline rapidly.

I have mentioned that I struggled massively after my surgery, knowing someone had invaded and been so intimate with my body. I needed to know what I had gone through and I did this by watching procedures and following other patient journeys.

Talking to many patients they all seem to have had some level of emotional stress.

Imagine buddies on the ward, there for patients and families who would like a chat or just a friendly face who has the time to invest and not tied down by workload as the healthcare professionals are.

Imagine consultants having access to their own team of buddies who can mentor their patients right from the start of the journey to motivate the patient to get physically and emotionally ready prior to the procedure.

Imagine turning the ward day room into a fantastic interactive, bright, cheerful, even inspirational arena/studio, where buddies can go and spend time with patients to watch a fun movie or play an uplifting interactive game or just having a one to one chat.

Imagine pioneering a unique approach, backed up by independent scientific evidence of the positive benefits, where the system can be rolled out to all cardiac centres around the world.

Two more patients, Alma and Lillian, were kind enough to tell me their stories.

Patient Alma – Her story

I first met Alma when I had been interviewing Tony Walker. He introduced me to her and said she was interested in the Buddy Beat concept I was hoping to develop. I met Alma a few days later in Costa Coffee in the hospital foyer to hear her story.

Alma's story starts around 2004, when she had her first heart attack. She was at work and had terrible chest pain. After three days, it got so severe that she went to see her doctor. He sent her up to A&E immediately. An angiogram was organised which showed Alma had an occluded coronary artery which they were able to resolve with medication.

Three years later, Alma had another heart attack. This time they treated it with coronary angioplasty which is a minimally invasive procedure carried out by a cardiologist (not a surgeon) in a catheter lab. A balloon attached to a wire is first inserted into one of the arteries in your groin, your wrist, or your arm. The wire is then carefully guided towards the site of the blockage in your coronary artery and the balloon inflated to clear the blockage. Sometimes another device called a stent is left in place to keep the artery open. When the cardiologist subsequently deflates the balloon, the stent stays in place to help blood flow.

Seven years on and Alma had her third heart attack. This time she was admitted, and another angiogram found that she now had three very badly blocked arteries. Within two weeks, she had an appointment to meet Mr Walker. After his assessment, he advised Alma that she was at risk of experiencing another incident, one which could be fatal. Her coronary artery disease had developed to the point where she would require surgery. And Alma's response? She is a grown woman, so if Mr Walker would take the risk then she would agree to treatment. Two weeks later, she got the call.

Alma remembers that though her recovery was horrendous, and she was burdened with many obstacles, she was happy to go through it if it meant getting better. Eventually, Alma went home and joined the rehab programme but unfortunately couldn't finish it due to her other health issues.

Alma is not a lady who will be climbing Kilimanjaro anytime soon or running a marathon. What she does represent are the many individuals who can, following surgery, resume everyday tasks such as climbing stairs and pushing a trolley around a supermarket. It is perhaps easy to take such things for granted, that is until we lose our ability to do them. Alma now has a much better quality of life.

What is most impressive is the change in her emotional state and her new attitude to tackling challenges. Before she would question whether she could do certain tasks, now she just gets on and does them. She says she feels on top of the world and hasn't felt this good for many, many years. Alma is sure this is all down to Blackpool Victoria Hospital's Cardiac Centre and, most of all, her consultant, Mr Walker.

Meeting Alma shows me how patient-consultant relationships can become very intense. It is no small thing for somebody to give you your life back and without Mr Walker's intervention, Alma would have probably died.

Alma calls Mr Walker her 'Superman'. She adores him. She has even presented him with an engraved mug with 'The Best Surgeon in the World' on it. I asked Mr Bose if he had ever had a similar relationship with a patient. He told me of a six-foot-four male rugby player who gave him a bear hug that lasted what seemed like a lifetime.

In all the consultant's offices, the walls and shelves are covered in thank-you cards and gifts from patients who have been given their life back.

Alma, without any provocation by me, also praised the CICU and ward staff, highlighting their incredible dedication to caring for their patients. I must admit I would have to agree with her on this. I also felt their commitment to care was well beyond the call of duty.

Alma has now joined the many former patients who have become volunteers at the hospital as a way of saying thank you and giving something back.

Lilian was another patient who was happy to share her journey:

Patient Lilian - Her story

I first met Lilian when I sat in on one of Mr Bose's clinics. Lilian and her husband Geoff wanted more clarification on the procedure she was about to undertake in a week's time. Mr Bose, in his light-hearted but professional manner, helped them understand the process and the potential outcomes.

Lilian was born during the war in a small village in the Yorkshire Dales. She grew up near her grandmother who used to love playing the piano. She taught Lilian how to play.

In her teens, the family emigrated to Victoria, Australia where Lilian acquired a degree in music. Throughout the time she was in Australia, there were no jobs for a pianist, so she took a job as a teacher to earn some money.

On a holiday in England, she was pleased to find that there was a demand for pianists working with concert groups, choirs, and theatre groups. Lilian started to work with a variety of organisations as a jobbing pianist. She even did a panto season. 'Oh yes she did.'

The time came when she realised, she needed a proper job and so Lilian became a teacher in Hackney, London. While working at the Hackney school, she began experiencing chest pains and soon found herself attending the London Chest Hospital. It was there they determined that she had atrial fibrillation (AF) for which she was prescribed medication.

During walks in the Alps and the Lake District, Lilian noticed she was becoming increasingly lethargic. She hardly wanted to walk far, and much preferred a trip to a coffee shop. Back home she was put on a twenty-hour heart monitor which confirmed her AF. The symptoms steadily worsened and, following an echocardiogram, she was diagnosed as having aortic stenosis. Sometime later, Lilian underwent another round of tests and her cardiologist felt it was time to refer her to a cardiac surgeon.

Now, Lilian had a choice of two surgeons, Mr Bose being one of them. As a musician, she associated the name 'Bose' with superior speakers and so made her choice. Very scientific Lilian!

Lilian is a very perceptive person. On meeting Mr Bose for the first time, she noticed he was dressed in a very sharp suit with a pink tie and thought, "He's trying to make an impression." Something else she noticed was that as he was talking, he was looking at her, noticing her reactions to what he was saying. Lilian was concerned about the safety of open-heart surgery. Mr Bose assured the pair that he would always do the utmost to return Lilian to Geoff safely. Lilian appreciated his sense of humour. As she put it, he had a sparkle. She says he was very easy to speak to and straight with the answers to her questions.

Lilian would have a replacement aortic valve, ablation, and a left atrial appendage. The initial period following surgery wasn't as smooth as she had hoped. Lillian experienced several bouts of AF, even being readmitted to the hospital via ambulance.

Since then, however, Lilian has returned to walking the fells.

Having been privileged to have undertaken this journey I have come to the conclusion that the patient journey can be broken down into three easily definable phases. These are the phases and my views on how they could be managed:

Phase 1. Pre-Operative - The period that covers the initial diagnosis and the consultations with the cardiac professionals. The realisation of the situation for the patient and the need to get them physically and emotionally prepared for the procedure

- With the first consultant clinic letter, a Buddy Beat booklet should be included with a number of social media sites for them to visit to gain some level of knowledge and understanding of their potential journey. Also, the booklet would request them to respond as to whether they would like to be part of the Buddy Beat programme.

- All clinic waiting areas are anything but inspiring, especially when you are there for an extended amount of time due to 'overrunning' clinics. One side of the waiting room should be converted into a more private area where the consultant patients on the Buddy Beat programme are taken to watch relevant videos and meet Buddies prior to their consultation.

- Personally, I believe this would be an uplifting experience (in relative terms) and create a much more positive environment prior to the consultation.

- When called into the consultation, it would hope this would progress much quicker as the patient has some knowledge and understands some of the terminology saving consultant time.

- Once the prognosis is known, then a personalised pre-op mentoring programme is developed with the inclusion of the rehab team to get the patient emotionally and physically ready for the procedure.

- Same-day admissions would have the patient's Buddy or an 'On-Call' Buddy for any patient needing moral support at this point. Those second on the list will have an opportunity to listen to music, watch a movie etc or just sit with their family. This idea is all based around a belief that the bodies vital organs will respond better to the trauma of the anaesthetic drugs and physical turmoil if in a relaxed state.

Phase 2. The procedure and hospitalisation - The critical period of surgery and initial stages of recovery.

- At this hospitalisation stage, the patient is the capable hands of the health care professionals.

- Their Buddy or the 'On Call' Buddy would be there as a friendly face when they come around. The Buddy will stay with them and talk to their family throughout their hospital stay.

Phase 3. Post Procedure - The post-surgery element that mainly takes place at home.

- Again, in partnership with the rehab team, a personalised programme will be developed to help them over the first few weeks at home. As well as the physical checks Buddies will be checking for any signs of emotional concern.

- The length of the Buddy involvement will be directly related to the progress made and the desire of the patient and family to continue the mentoring.

- Testing and evaluation will take place at key stages of the process and logged for 'crunching' at a later date.

Thirty years ago, heart surgery was all about the plumbing. Medication and physio have now become core to cardiac rehab, but what is still missing is the inclusion of the emotional wellbeing of the patient. Hopefully, it won't be too long before this is seen as a critical phase of the overall wellbeing and recovery of the patient.

The message I would like to champion is that heart surgery gives you the chance of a 'Second Life', a realisation that life is there to be lived and enjoyed for the time we have it.

Reader Question

You have been given a second chance in life.

What is the first thing you want to achieve with your new given opportunity?

Chapter 8

Laughter in the Face of Trauma

**Laughter is the greatest therapy we have,
yet we use it the least.**

So, you've just been told you have a life-
threatening illness, nothing funny about that.
Suddenly laughing and having fun seem to be at
the other end of life's spectrum.

I have on many occasions sat in the waiting
room of the Lancashire Cardiac Centre. Watching
patients as they wait for their consultation with
their doctor or consultant. I can confirm there was
very little frivolity happening there.

However, have you ever thought how
powerful laughter is as a therapy?

Legend has it that shortly after Adam was
created, he complained:

*'O, Lord! You have given the lion fierce teeth and
claws, and the elephant formidable tusks; you have given
the deer swiftness of legs, and the turtle a protective
shell; you have given the birds of flight wings, but you
have left me altogether defenceless.' And the Lord said
unto Adam: 'I have given you an invisible weapon, one
that will serve you and your children better than any
weapons of fight or flight, a quality that will save you,
even from yourself. I have given you .... 'a sense of
humour.'*

We are defenceless without humour. If we fail
to see the irony in our circumstances, the situation

may appear dispiriting. Laughter is a way of 'thumbing one's nose' at the inescapable and incomprehensible vagaries of existence, declaring, 'I choose to rise above this. I choose to meet life head-on.' Laughter is freedom.

Laughter can actually improve your health. It's official: laughter is scientifically recognised as a very strong medication. It draws people together in ways that trigger healthy physical and emotional changes in the body. Laughter strengthens your immune system, boosts mood, diminishes pain, and protects you from the damaging effects of stress.

As children, we laugh hundreds of times a day. Even as babies, we smile long before we say our first word. But as an adult life tends to get more serious and laughter more infrequent.

Laughter is a powerful antidote to stress, pain, and conflict. Nothing works faster or more dependably to bring your mind and body back into balance than a good laugh. Humour lightens your burdens, inspires hope, connects you to others. It also helps you to release anger and be more forgiving.

With so much power to heal and renew, the ability to laugh easily and frequently is a tremendous resource for surmounting both physical and emotional health. Best of all, this priceless medicine is fun, free, and easy to use.

It triggers the release of endorphins, the body's natural feel-good chemicals. Endorphins promote an overall sense of well-being and can even relieve pain.

Laughter may even help you to live longer. A study in Norway found that people with a strong sense of humour outlived those who didn't laugh as much. The difference was particularly notable for those battling cancer or heart disease.

Another research programme that would endorse this was done by Dr Lee Berk in the US. Dr Berk and his team from the psycho-neuro-immunology department did a study on the physical impact of laughter. In one study, heart-attack patients were divided into two groups; one half was placed under standard medical care with medication while being left to their own devices. The other half watched humorous videos for thirty minutes a day.

After one year, the results showed the group that had watched the humorous videos had fewer arrhythmias, lower blood pressure, lower levels of stress hormones, and required lower levels of medication. The non-humour group had two and a half times more recurrent heart-attacks.

In the late sixties, there was a young American man called Hunter Adams. Hunter always wanted to be a doctor but not necessarily the stereotypical doctor. In his early days, Hunter suffered from mental illness and entered a mental institution. Here he met the wealthy businessman and philanthropist Arthur Mendleson. Arthur would hold up four fingers and ask inmates how many fingers they saw. Most would answer four.

One day, Hunter sheepishly entered Arthur's room and asked him, "What's the answer to the four-finger question?" Again, Arthur held up four fingers and said, "What do you see?" With a big frown on his face, Hunter whispered, "Six." Brilliant came the response from Arthur, "Don't see what you can see, see what you can't see."

During the chat, Hunter noticed the paper cup with Arthur's tea in it was leaking. Hunter found a bit of sticky tape and stuck it to the cup. Arthur looked up and said from now on you will be known as 'Patch'.

Patch went to medical school but was frustrated with the fact he would not have any contact with patients until the third year. Patch was all about the patients and had a very strong vision of how they should be cared for.

He was a bit of a maverick and got up to all sorts of mischief. One day, he got hold of a white coat, which doctors wore back then and joined a 3rd year group of students on their ward round with a doctor.

On arrival at the end of a patient bed, the doctor started to recite in a rather loud voice the patients' full medical history. Some of the students asked specific questions about her condition and what the doctor had prescribed. From the back of the group, Patch was heard to say, "Does the patient have a name, Sir?"

In another of Patch's maverick moments, he again dressed up in a white coat and toured the wards. He found himself in a children's cancer ward. The children were all very quiet, lying on their backs, some with chemotherapy drips attached.

Patch asked one of them their name, at the same time, he noticed a red sphere on the table next to the bed. In a moment of madness, he split the sphere and put it on his nose and started acting like a red-nosed clown. The child burst out laughing. Then Patch put a rubber glove on his head and started clucking like a chicken suddenly all the kids on the ward were laughing uncontrollably. He then put a bedpan on his head and two on his feet and started to act as a man possessed. From being very quiet and sombre when Patch walked in, the children were now in hysterics.

Patch was in big trouble. He was summoned by the University Dean. The Dean said to him, "You have a brilliant mind Adams but like many people with brilliant minds, they don't think the rules apply to them." He continued to say patients don't need a friend or a clown, they need a doctor. Patch replied, "Treat the disease and sometimes you win, sometimes you lose. Treat the person and you win every time, Sir."

In one of Patch's university reports, it said 'This man suffers from excessive happiness.'

Patch continued to develop his clown theme for hospitals and can now boast over one thousand clowns around the world going into hospitals to spread laughter, the 'Patch Adams' way.

Patch also took the humour into his real passion which was to set up a free hospital where he would carry out his vision of treating the patient, not the illness and all for free. He called it the Gesundheit Institute. Gesundheit in German means 'bless you' something we often say when people sneeze.

Patch Adams became and still is, a phenomenon within American healthcare. Partly so, by the 1998 Hollywood blockbuster based on his life. In the film, Robin Williams played the role of Patch.

If you have never seen the movie, you must; it's extremely thought-provoking and incredibly inspirational.

I had a little part to play in the development of this movie as my brother-in-law lives in San Francisco and ran an art gallery and framing business back in the late 90s. Unfortunately, his son Danny who was only little at the time had been diagnosed with leukaemia and was receiving treatment in a downtown San Francisco hospital.

Helen and I with our three kids were visiting at the time, helping Mike and Patty out with the emotional turmoil and stresses of having to cope with such a traumatic situation.

On the day in question, Helen and Patty had gone to the hospital, Mike and I had called in at the framing shop in downtown San Francisco. Whilst at the shop, Mike received a call from Patty saying, "Get over here right away as the Hollywood actor Robin Williams is on the ward with a clown and is soon to be with Danny."

Mike drove across the city as if our lives depended on it. We had many single-digit fingers waved at us as we cut up so many drivers to get to the hospital as quickly as possible. We ran up the stairs to the ward, burst in and found Danny all wired up to his chemotherapy drip but in fits of laughter, as the clown and Robin Williams were going through a routine. Fortunately, Helen and Patty had told them we were on the way, so he and the clown stayed until we got there.

Robin and the clown stayed with Danny for ages. We were fortunate to have a chat with the late, great Robin Williams and got the mandatory autograph. We found out Robin Williams and the clown, which we later found out to be Patch, were doing research for the movie.

For days after, Danny and indeed all of us, were in great spirits thanks to the visit which again endorses the fact that humour and uplifting experiences have a massive effect on your emotional and physical wellbeing.

I have written to Patch whilst writing the book. You can only communicate directly with Patch by sending him a letter by post. He doesn't use a computer or any kind of technology. I wrote to him on a concept I am setting up called 'Buddy Beat'. I tracked the letter on-line and watched its progression to Patch. I was elated when the tracking showed it had finally got to its destination.

I was even more elated when a mere three days later, a big brown Jiffy bag arrived from the US. Inside was a signed copy of his book and a personal hand-written letter. Within it, Patch had written, 'Everyone needs a buddy, especially when they are ill.' He also invited me to join him on a clown outreach programme in Morocco. A clown outreach is where Patch and a group of volunteers dress up as clowns and visit hospitals and orphanages to spread a little joy. Unfortunately, the timings did not fit for me, but I do plan to join him on an outreach programme in Russia.

There is a mistaken belief that since the medical profession is a serious one, doctors should appear intense, sincere and solemn, but definitely not flippant. Too many people confuse seriousness with professionalism so put a lid on humour. They think joking would render the doctor's behaviour unprofessional.

I believe that Mr Bose, my consultant surgeon, understands the power of humour in stressful situations. I have shadowed him in theatre and sat in on his clinics, with patients who are obviously worried about their health and the future. Mr Bose is a master of assessing the situation and bringing humour into a consultation when he feels it will help the situation.

In the book *The Anatomy of an Illness,* Norman Cousins first called the attention of the medical community to the potential therapeutic effects of humour when he described his utilisation of laughter during treatment for his own ankylosing spondylitis (arthritis of the spine).

Believing that negative emotions had an adverse impact on his health, he theorised that positive emotions would have a positive effect. He believed that the experience of laughter could open him up to feelings of joy, hope, confidence and love. 'If you can laugh at it, you can survive it.'

'Even if laughter produces no specific biochemical changes,' according to Norman Cousins, 'it accomplishes one very essential purpose. It tends to block deep feelings of anxiety, fear and even panic that frequently accompany serious illness. It helps free the body of the constricting effects of the negative emotions that in turn may impair the healing system.' According to Cousins personal experience, ten minutes of laughter resulted in two hours of pain-free sleep.

Research has shown that laughter has an anti-inflammatory effect that protects blood vessels and heart muscles from the damaging effects of cardiovascular disease. How this happens isn't entirely understood, but it seems related to lessening the body's stress response, which is directly linked to increased inflammation.

I believe regular, hearty laughter should be identified as just as important as a physical intervention and medication in healthcare.

But what's the difference between humour and jokes. See if you laugh at this old Groucho Marks joke.

"Yesterday, I shot an Elephant in my pyjama's...how he got in them I have no idea."

Some people will have found it funny, others may not. Some may even question if a joke about shooting Elephants is politically incorrect in today's PC society.

Or how about this one:

"Two American hunters are in a forest; one collapses on the ground. The other calls 911 to say his mate has just collapsed and he thinks he's dead. The operator responds "can you make sure he's dead" the operator hears a gunshot. The man returned to the phone and confirmed: "he's definitely dead."

Here are a couple of hospital jokes:

"After having heart surgery, a male patient is about to leave the hospital and asks his consultant, "Can I start having sex" to which the consultant whispered "of course! but only with your wife, we don't want you getting too excited."

Or

"Nurse Sandra, an attractive woman, took her problem to the hospital staff psychiatrist where she worked. "Doctor, you must help me," she pleaded. "It's got to a stage where every time I date one of the young doctors, I end up sleeping with him and then afterwards, I feel guilty and depressed for a week." "I see," nodded the psychiatrist. "And you, want me to give you the will power to stop this happening?" "NO!!!" exclaimed the nurse. "I want you to fix it, so I won't feel guilty and depressed afterwards!"

Gallows, or black humour, is a term to cover the humour created from the darker side of traumatic events that produce jokes on the subject. No matter how devastating or traumatic an event is, within minutes of it happening, the internet is full of gallows humour and jokes on the incident.

In World War 1, probably the most horrendous situation and environment the human body and spirit has ever had to endure, soldiers used a lot of gallows humour to help them survive.

To the ordinary soldier, humour and especially black humour was as essential as their rifle and bayonet for survival. It was a defensive weapon, vital to staving off the descent into insanity that was the logical reaction to the surrounding hell they found themselves in.

TV comedy programmes such as *Dad's Army* and *Blackadder* used the gallows humour of war.

Another period of history where Black humour can be seen as a coping mechanism is the Holocaust. When survivors were asked how they survived such atrocities, interviewers were taken back when the answer they got was humour and laughter.

Black, or gallows humour, has long been recognised as having therapeutic value, particularly when used by individuals dealing with traumatic incidents. With this in mind, it is no surprise that this type of humour is commonly used by emergency services personnel. It is a bona fide coping mechanism which can contribute to the resilience, health and wellbeing of emergency services personnel but one which, to the uninitiated, may appear callous and uncaring.

So, what is *Comic Relief* in a trauma environment? Apart from being a very successful British charity, It's a humorous interlude into a tragedy or a traumatic experience. It takes you away from the reality of a devastating or traumatic situation and brings a moment of 'comic relief'.

Let's start with William Shakespeare. Shakespeare was a master of comic relief and frequently incorporated comedy elements into many of his plays. He often used a clownish, bumbling type of fool to provide it. Let's look at a prominent example in a Shakespearean tragedy.

In Act II: Scene 3 of Macbeth', the drunken porter (gatekeeper at Macbeth's castle) is a buffoon who appears between the horrific murder of King Duncan and the gruesome discovery of his body. He imagines he is the gatekeeper of hell, and his hallucinations are delivered with enough slapstick, dirty jokes, and vulgarities to keep the audience in stitches. After this, the horror of King Duncan's butchered corpse is magnified for the audience.

In an interview I did with a couple of secretaries to the consultants, one of them told of a telephone conversation she had with a patient enquiring about his life-threatening procedure date. The conversation went something like this:

'Patient; "Sorry I keep phoning you up"

Secretary: "It's fine, at least we know you're still with us"

Obviously, the secretary was devastated when she realised what she had said. Fortunately, the patient saw the funny side and mentioned it every time they phoned after the event. A great example of real-life comic relief.

Humour is an integral part of human relationships and plays numerous and significant roles in both our personal and social lives. Theories on humour abound and come from a wide variety of perspectives such as psychological, sociological, anthropological, linguistic and theatrical.

It is accepted that humour can act as a form of tension release and as mentioned above, can be used as a valuable coping strategy for those who have to encounter unpleasant or traumatic events such as life-threatening illness or even death.

Plato and Aristotle contemplated the meaning of comedy while laying the foundations of Western philosophy. Charles Darwin looked for the seeds of laughter in the joyful cries of tickled chimpanzees. Sigmund Freud sought the underlying motivations behind jokes in the nooks and crannies of our unconscious minds.

Humour, I believe, is the by-product of circumstance, whereas a joke is a response to a short story or one-liner.

Getting a laugh is a subtle and complicated business. Any professional comedian knows the same joke can work one night and flop the next. There's a long queue of public figures who will vouch for the cost of misjudged humour. Take Gerald Ratner, the managing director of Ratners the one-time retail jewellery giant. He wiped £500 million off the value of his family jewellery business and lost his £650,000 salary in 1991 because a joke backfired. To get a laugh, he said that a £4.95 cut-glass sherry decanter with six glasses on a silver-plated tray was, "Total crap" and went on to say that the earrings in his shops were cheaper than a prawn sandwich and probably wouldn't last as long.

Genuine humour requires us to read the context of a situation, pick the right tone, and choose our pauses. A good friend of mine was the managing director of a radio station chain. At a presenter conference, he said I could give you a joke to use on the radio. Some of you would get a laugh from it and some of you wouldn't. It's all in the delivery and timing.

Comedians like Michael McIntyre, Peter Kay and Lee Evans can fill 20,000-seater stadiums because people want to relieve themselves from the stresses of life and work. Being with many likeminded people in the same arena just seems to up the excitement and positive response to the comedian's jokes. These guys have mastered the psychology of delivery and timing. Audiences leaving their concerts are uplifted, happy and feel mentally and physically rejuvenated for the experience.

What fascinates me is a comedian can only tell a joke once. For example, if a comedian tells a joke for the first time, the response is spontaneous and heartfelt. However, if they were to use the same joke again in the same show, the response would be heavily diminished and if they chose to use it a third and fourth time, the laughter would become non-existent.

That reminds me of my youth when I had a white Dansett record player. Dansett were state of the art back then as you could load up the vinyl records on a spindle in the middle of the turntable. When one record finished, the next one would drop down and start to play. Back in those days, I only had a handful of records, so they were repeated over and over again. Every time I played them, I got less and less joy from the song, until I got fed up of hearing it. So, why do we get bored with hearing the same thing over and over again? Answers to chris@thisoldheartofmine.co.uk please.

Sometimes, no words are needed to make someone smile; a look is enough. Tommy Cooper was a genius at this. He didn't have to say anything to get an audience howling. Lee Evans is another. Lee can have an audience of 15,000 doubled up just by walking on to the stage.

Laughter doesn't always have a connection to humour. It can be nervous, as in job interviews, diplomatic, as in conversations with your boss. Fake to cover up when you haven't heard what someone said. In other words, it serves a multitude of social purposes. Robert Provine, a professor of psychology and neuroscience at the University of Maryland-Baltimore County, believes that laughter may have pre-dated human speech by millions of years, hardwiring it into the human brain in the process. The fact that laughter arrives well before speech for babies, and manifests in every culture, proves that it is an instinctive and universal mechanism. Why do babies seem to laugh when they don't have any reference as to what is funny?

Who laughs the most?

Studies by a neuroscientist at University College London, refer to laughter as an index of the strength of a relationship. They believe that mirroring another person's emotional state, through laughing, is a way of demonstrating affiliation and strengthening bonds. They found the person who laughs the most at any one time tends to be the person speaking rather than the one who's listening. This makes sense when we understand that laughter induces laughter in others. If you're not sure, here is a true story. BBC Radio 4 presenter Charlotte Green, whilst presenting the news played the earliest known recording of the human voice but got the giggles when a colleague whispered it sounded like a bee in a jar.

Charlotte could barely finish the news as she was in hysterics. Rather than making calls of protest for lowering the professional standards of the BBC, Listeners phoned in to report that Green's laughter had, 'Made their day.'

I remember when I was a child, I went to Blackpool on holiday and went to the pleasure beach. Within the amusement arcade was something called the 'Laughing Policeman.' This was a full-sized dummy dressed up as a policeman in a giant perspex cylinder. When you put sixpence (oh yes, I am going way back) in the slot, suddenly the policeman would start laughing. No matter how many times I visited, I always ended up in hysterics watching the policeman laugh.

So, it's a fact, every human being on the planet likes a laugh and more importantly, needs to laugh for health reasons. So, how can we use the therapeutic value in heart surgery? As a patient and trying to remember the time I spent in hospital during my first procedure, humour was not at the forefront of my mind or played any formal part in my recovery programme.

At the cardiac centre, patients tend to be predominately more mature than other areas of the hospital. So, is a clown coming in and messing around the answer? On the other hand, it may be the perfect time for a bit of fun. Patch Adams says he has made many people laugh on their death beds. What better way to pass on than with a smile on your face? It's worth thinking about.

The revered comedian Billy Connolly was diagnosed with the degenerative neurological Parkinson's disease. In a BBC documentary, Sir Billy reflects on his life and career in showbiz and insists he is not scared of death. In the documentary, he said, "Life, is slipping away and I can feel it and I should, I'm seventy-five. I'm near the end. I'm a damn sight nearer the end than I am the beginning (the circle of life). But it doesn't frighten me, it's an adventure and it is quite interesting to see myself slipping away."

"Bits slip off and leave me, talents and attributes are no longer there to draw from. I don't have the balance I used to have; I don't have the energy I used to have. I can't hear the way I used to hear; I can't see as good as I used to. I can't remember the way I used to remember. They all came one at a time and they all seem to be slipping away one at a time. It's like somebody who is in charge of you is saying, right Billy, I added all these bits when you were born, now it is time to take them back."

Speaking about Parkinson's, he said, "It takes a certain calm to deal with, and sometimes I don't have it. I sometimes get angry with it, but that doesn't last long, I just collapse in laughter."

I recently read that the most successful sector of the entertainment business is comedy, with a leading British comedian grossing considerably more than most 'A list' Hollywood actors. Surely, this shows that we all like a good laugh to help us escape from the stresses and pressures of everyday life even if it is for a short period of time.

Most cardiac wards have what is called a day room, its purpose is supposedly a quiet place where patient and family can go for some privacy. That said, most of the day rooms I have visited seem to be very uninspiring, extremely unwelcoming even depressing. I have yet to see anyone using them. Yes, they have a few chairs in them that are well past their sell-by date and maybe a fourteen-inch TV in the corner but there is nothing in these rooms to lift the emotional well-being of the patients. Nothing to lift the spirits and motivation of patients and family members.

I have a crazy idea for these rooms, that in my humble opinion, would transform them into a mainstream strand of patients' rehabilitation. What about if we transformed the room from a room that no-one uses to one that is inspirational, uplifting and empowering? Why couldn't it have a large flat screen on a wall with lots of fun movies to watch? What about covering the walls with fun images and jokes guaranteed to make everyone smile?

Just as patients are urged to do a certain amount of physiotherapy a day whilst on the ward, why not the same commitment with laughter and humour? We know everyone on the planet needs the stimulation and health benefits of laughter and from scientific research, we know laughter is good for us both mentally and physically, why isn't it part of mainstream healthcare?

Patch Adam's had a Hollywood movie made about his belief in the health benefits of laughter. What other areas of medicine have had a Hollywood blockbuster made on it.

Reader Question

Count how many times you laugh in a day.

What could you do that would make you laugh more each day?

Chapter 9

Female Pioneers of Change

If you want to fly, let go of everything that weighs you down

Although this chapter has little reference to mine and other patients' journeys, it was one I really wanted to explore and highlight.

The chapter is quite controversial and opens up a whole minefield of potential conflict. My reason for including it in the book was not to promote Girl Power or to knock it but to explore women in what might be considered by some as a male frontier.

The Spice Girls, a cultural phenomenon in the 90's would probably lay claim to the rise of 'Girl Power'. However, twenty years earlier, an Australian singer by the name of Helen Reddy sang a song called 'I Am Women' which reached number one in the charts across the world. The first verse went like this;

> *I am woman, hear me roar*
> *In numbers too big to ignore*
> *And I know too much to go back and pretend*
> *Cause I've heard it all before*
> *And I've been down there on the floor*
> *No one's ever gonna keep me down again*

Another reason for this chapter was to give a balanced view of the reality that exists with woman at the top level of the NHS and other professions. At nurse and admin-level, the workforce is 95% female. But as you go up the ladder of responsibility, it becomes very much, a male domain. I wanted to explore why this was.

If my surgeon happened to be female or the airline pilot flying the plane to my holiday destination was female that would be fine with me. I believe the system or the people who do the recruiting would not put themselves at risk let alone the patients or the passengers by employing incompetent people.

For this chapter, I went outside the cardiac centre and interviewed people within business sectors that have some parallels with cardiothoracic surgery.

At the Lancashire Cardiac Centre, the Divisional Director at the time of writing; responsible for some 1,500 people, was Dr Helen Saunders. Dr Saunders is also one of the department's top anaesthetists. Dr Saunders is not a power dresser, nor does she have that aggression that you see in some powerful businesswomen. Dr Saunders is a quietly spoken woman who understands how to manage situations in a calm and controlled way which has served her well in what could be considered as a strong testosterone dominated department.

At the time of doing my research, the department had two female registrar surgeons.

Female cardiothoracic surgeons account for about 3% of their profession, similar to that of female airline pilots worldwide. Yet amongst dentists and vets, females make up in excess of 50%. It begs the question, why?

I can understand the vet scenario because female love of pets starts at a very early age, so it's easy to see where their love of wanting to become a vet comes from.

That said, the Yorkshire TV Vet James Heriot in his checked shirt, tartan jacket, walking trousers, balding head and public-school voice, created a stereotype of what a Vet should look and sound like. It did nothing to help the female cause.

One young female vet I spoke to was confronted by a man with a dog that had a twisted gut. Unfortunately, I know from a sad episode with Barny our agility Labrador that a twisted gut is both a serious, complicated and a painful condition for any dog to experience.

When the young vet explained that the dog needed an emergency operation the man asked if there was a male vet who could perform the operation, as he didn't want a female to operate on his dog.

Another young vet wearing minimal make-up was asked directly by a male dog owner whether makeup was appropriate for a vet.

One thing I have never understood though, whether you are a male or a female, is why you would want to be a dentist.

So, if the number of women vets and dentists exceed 50%, how come the level of female heart surgeons and airline pilots are as low as 3%?

I need to research the parallels, if any, between female airline pilots and female cardiac surgeons. I wanted to get their views on their journeys.

I contacted the British Women Pilots' Association (BWPA) and asked if I could get an interview with a couple of airline pilots. An advert was put on the website and a number of pilots were happy to give me an interview. I picked those I thought would give me a balanced view of life within their profession, so I chose a retired 747 training captain, a pilot with strong views on the subject and a current captain flying the latest Boeing Dreamliner. Between them, I hoped to get a balanced overview. What I did get is very differing views of the same journey.

Sarah is a pilot who provided her story, written in her own words.

Pilot Sarah – Her story

I grew up in Sussex and Kent, went to a Grammar school. I left school (and home!) at 16. Went to work with horses - show jumpers and racehorses. At 17, I changed direction. My neighbour ran a gliding club and I started working for her. She taught me to glide. At the time, I didn't even know what a glider was, knew nothing about planes and hadn't thought about being a pilot. I had wanted to be a vet at school, but the career adviser didn't think so and sent me to Mothercare for my week's work experience.

At 18, I moved to America to work with horse vets and after a year went travelling.

On my return to the UK, I contacted the big gliding clubs in the UK and got a couple of job offers. I ended up working in the office at Booker Gliding Club in 1990.

I saw lots of airline pilots, who seemed to have far too much money and time off, go gliding. 99% were male.

Being a pilot seemed like a good job! So, I worked there in the 1990s. I started thinking about doing my PPL.

Every flight school was so sexist. They would ignore me, ask if I was buying a present for my boyfriend. If I went with my boyfriend, I would get ignored. Even though he had no intention of flying, they would talk to him.

Around 1991, I got fifteen hours scholarship with the Air League. My instructor was very much in it for himself, he wanted to get the instrument and cross-country hours so instead of training me to my first solo flight, I ended up doing instrument and cross-country flights in poor weather and not learning much.

In 1994, I decided to give it another go. I was already a glider pilot but went to San Diego to do an intensive PPL course. I was there for 3.5 weeks and got it done. It was a fabulous time, great instructor, and team, very much work hard play hard. I was very much "one of the boys" out drinking and playing pool most nights! From then on, I went back for various holidays to do further ratings and eventually my FAA ATP. I converted everything to CAA and started to look for a job.

By this point I was broke. I had lived in a caravan for a year, bought a house, had a car I got for £100 that conked out every time it rained. I had lodgers to pay the bills.

I applied to CTC Aviation who were new at the time. I passed all their assessment (at the time only about 5% got through). I was offered a job with a small airline, Leisure International on the Airbus, subject to interview. The timescale was short, I think we heard on the Wednesday, flew to Johannesburg on Friday to start an intensive 4-week course!! Usually, it would be around eight weeks and you'd get all the study material in advance!

So, off we went to the interview, two men; two women. We were met by one of their top guys, a Captain. He looked us up and down and his first words to us were "bloody hell, two women!" Honestly, they were his exact words!! Never forgotten!

So, we were like 'wow' what are we getting in to here! And this was 1998 in the UK so not that long ago! Anyway, we got the job, went to Africa for our training and four weeks later, got our type ratings.

We were issued with men's uniforms as that's all they had: Suit and tie.

Uniforms have always been an issue. Earlier on you could only have 29" inside leg in women's trousers. That was it. I am tall so this didn't work! They got me some unhemmed ones and told me to sort it myself.

Another time, the uniform we got consisted of cabin crew jacket, trousers, cabin crew scarf, pilot shirt.

Anyway, we all trundled along.

Many people back then told female pilots they only got the job as a nod to equality. I always pointed out that they must think the male selectors were stupid if they were picking pilots who couldn't do the job.

I remember being on a crew bus to the plane. The Captain turned to me; looked me up and down and said, "Oh I've never flown with a female pilot before" in a disdainful voice. "And you probably won't want to fly with one again after a day with me," I quipped back.

In the old days, we had flight deck visits. One old chap came in and was quite rude to me, then turned his back to me (I was actually the one flying) and said in a haughty voice to the male Captain, "Oh, they let women fly now do they?" and the Captain, a lovely guy, and a training captain, came straight back at him, and said,

"Yes, since the war. Sarah is one of the best pilots I've flown with actually." The passenger didn't like that!!

I've also had a male passenger get on and seeing me said, "Oh! I'm not flying with a female pilot! You'll need to get a proper pilot in!" The cabin crew, who always supported me, said, "Oh sir, well today we have two female pilots because the Captain is female too". He still wanted me removed or he wouldn't fly, so I said, "Shall we start looking for your bags Sir? Because this flight is going and if you don't wish to travel, we can offload you." Funnily enough, he flew with us.

We often had issues in places like Cyprus and Turkey. In Cyprus, the ground agents would talk to any male staff member about pilot paperwork, even if they were cabin crew. One night in Paphos, I remember the agent came in, saw me, looked to my left, saw the female Captain, he left the flight deck and asked the cabin crew where the men were. The senior cabin crew member told him that it was an all-female crew. "There is no responsible male on board?" he exclaimed, shocked.

Overall, most male pilots are fine. We used to have the odd leery one who would stare at your chest or want to touch you, but most have gone.

Cabin crews have been fab, always telling me I do the smoothest landings and supporting me in front of passengers.

Passengers still to this day will say, "Well done" or "Well done for getting us here" or "Oh, did you fly this" or "When will you get to fly it?" (usually after I've just landed them in a stonking crosswind or difficult approach). The men go on about parking and reversing. Or say, "Not bad. For a woman." I say, "Oh, are you a pilot?"

One man told me he thought the landing was rubbish. It was, in my view, and that of the cabin crew, an extremely smooth landing. So, he obviously had decided to say that just because I was a woman.

No one ever says, "Well done" to the men!

To anyone female coming into flying or becoming surgeons, I would tell them they need a thick skin, a good sense of humour, and be able to keep your mouth shut when colleagues and public are rude to you!

Judith is a retired airline pilot who was also happy to share her story.

Pilot Judith – Her story

Judith recalls how Belfast was very grim when she was growing up there. The seventies were the worst decade for indiscriminate bombings. There were curfews, security fences, sirens and helicopters always hovering. There was a constant feeling of worry for loved ones. It's just how life was, and you got used to it.

Her parents were a Bank Manager and a teacher. So, Judith had the best upbringing possible in such a troubled city.

Apart from an occasional trip to the airport with her dad to see the planes, Judith's early passion was with horses. She left school without any real direction. Just obsessed with horses.

She trained as a nurse but quickly realised that was a big mistake, however, she completed her training. Whilst working as a nurse, she started to learn to fly. Her 'Eureka' moment came when she was nineteen and the wheels of the Cessna 150 she was learning in left the ground for the first time. That was the moment she realised this was what she wanted to do.

In the late seventies and early eighties, aviation was in a bad way: Laker had gone bankrupt, there were no airlines recruiting new pilots. The air force didn't take on women pilots. However, Judith did find a route to achieve her goal. That was to build up your hours and become a flying instructor.

Build up more hours so you can take the commercial pilots test and get a commercial licence. If you were lucky, you would get a job with an airline to build up more hours and then take the airline transport licence and move on. A long process, no matter whether you were male or female. Men, of course, could have joined the air force.

Judith spent a year getting her Private Pilot's Licence, another year building up the hours and getting the instructors rating. It took another two years getting an instructor's job and then working flat out to get in the hours.

In 1983, she went to navigation school in London with trips to Bournemouth to do the flying. This again was all self-funded. She sold a very valuable show jumping horse which she kept as an emergency fund ...her pilot training, she considered an emergency. She did get a grant from the Belfast Education Library Board to do the ground exams.

Judith admits she was quite a confident lady and in 1984, she contacted all the tiny airlines, large air taxi companies and the bigger airlines including Air UK, based in Norwich, who flew the Shorts 330, an ugly aircraft built in Judith's hometown of Belfast.

Because the training costs for the 330 were not huge, Air UK was prepared to take on pilots with the bare minimum of qualifications. Here, she broke through and got a job as a pilot. As Judith highlights, that first foot on *the ladder is the biggest breakthrough of any pilot's career. I assume it's the same in cardiac surgery.*

At this point, Judith says she was so focused on achieving her goal that she cannot remember encountering any male chauvinism at any stage although it probably did exist. When she did the training at Air UK, she was in a class of around thirty other pilots, three being female. She says everyone in the room had one clear objective and that was to become a commercial pilot... without becoming bankrupt.

As Judith recalls, life, relationships and communication were very different back then. There was a lot of banter between the pilots but nothing the females couldn't cope with or indeed respond to with a comment equal to any aimed at them.

All pilots in the eighties wanted to fly jets, so Air UK found it difficult to hold onto pilots. After two years, Judith moved on to DAN Air and flew the BAC 1-11. At this point, Dan-Air was only giving pilots a one-year contract, so as soon as you started with Dan-Air, you were looking for a new job. Judith's next job was with British Caledonian. Soon after joining, British Caledonian was bought out by British Airways as it was going bankrupt.

British Airways at that point had a massive recruitment drive for pilots across their entire fleet. So, Judith put in for the 747 having acquired the hours required by this stage. Now that came as a culture shock to the male BA pilots as they had never had a women pilot until then. Judith remembers a male pilot saying something very inappropriate in the crew room, but just accepted it and got on with the job.

Continuing Judith's journey, it took more than nine years before she became a captain; applying for all types of aircraft she thought she could become a captain on. She achieved this on the 757 and 767 which meant going back to short haul for a while.

Europe became her playground; she recalls this period as one of her happiest. She enjoyed being a captain and doing it how she thought it should be done. She believed everyone should get from A to B safely, they should have a laugh at least once or twice during the flight but again achieved in a very professional manner.

After a few years, Judith then became involved in recruitment, ground training and command development training, a highly innovative initiative from BA. They realised 1st officers were coming through to become Captains but not making the step up in their people management skills. Judith became influential in moulding the process for pilots of the future.

It was then time for her to return to the cockpit. This time it was the 747-400 and at the same time, the role of a training captain, a unique and prestigious role. This meant she was training and examining very senior pilots both from within BA and pilots coming in from other airlines.

In Judith's own words, "This was an amazing experience" as it took place in the simulator and in the air. Although today, all emergency procedures can be done in the simulator, the flying is just a normal operation check.

I explored the passenger reaction to having a woman pilot upfront. Judith said she had endless comments about women drivers. Like the other airline pilots interviewed, she had also experienced the situation of a man who wanted to get off because a woman was in control. BA used to encourage the pilot to stand at the door when passengers got off and some comments did get her down especially as women had been around since Orville and Wilber.

I asked Judith if she had any funny stories that she could repeat, she said there were many she couldn't repeat, (she did once we finished recording) but she does remember an incident where she was in the cockpit and two baggage trollies crashed into each other. Surprisingly, the police were called to the incident. The policemen came up to the flight deck and asked, 'Is this your aircraft madam?' just like they would if it were a car accident.

I wanted to get Judith's advice for young women who want to become airline pilots, cardiac surgeons or anything else in life. Her response was; she never saw herself as a woman, more a person with ambition and drive to achieve....an equal to anyone. Clearly, this was a great foundation for reaching the ultimate heights (excuse the pun) for Judith.

With those words of wisdom; reluctantly our interview concluded.

The third pilot kind enough to share her story was Ella.

Pilot Ella – Her story
Ella was born to parents who travelled due to her father being in the services. The fact that she moved around due to her fathers' postings meant she flew a lot and got an understanding of flying. She became fascinated in all aspects of aviation, airports, planes, fuelling, food, runways, she was interested in it all.

In school, she told the careers advisor she wanted to be an airline pilot. The advisor told her to apply to be an air stewardess (as they were known back then) but she was adamant she wanted to be a pilot. Fortunately, a teacher found an article in becoming a pilot and Ella was convinced she could do it.

At the age of 17, Ella had acquired her Private Pilot's Licence (PPL) which is no mean feat as it takes forty plus hours of flying and many classroom hours of learning the technical side of flight.

Ella decided university was not for her as she was completely focused and determined to become an airline pilot. She took a number of jobs to help fund her flying addiction. One of those jobs was a secretary for a small commercial airline that flew Piper Aztecs. In her spare time, she would fly with them.

She built up her hours to the point that she became a flying instructor, that led to her first commercial flying job; flying turboprops. From there, she joined the airline she has been with ever since and is now a captain on the Boeing 787 Dreamliner taking holidaymakers to some of the World's most exotic locations.

Ella is very softly spoken; however, it didn't take long to realise this is a lady who was always going to achieve her objective. She exudes a steely determination and the calmness you want in someone in control of 260 tons of aeroplane 35,000 feet in the air with you in the back.

When asked if she found it difficult making it in what could be perceived as a male-dominated industry, she replied: "I just became one of the boys."

Ella walked me through 'a day in the life of a pilot' so I could identify if there were any parallels with cardiac surgeons. The process went something like this. Pilots would arrive at the crew room one hour before departure. Prior to this, they may have downloaded all the flight details such a flight plan, number of passengers, fuel load, weather from home. If not, this will be done on arrival at the crew room. The parallel with the cardiac surgeon is they also acquire all the info they need for the patient such as looking at the patient's angiogram, the patient notes for things like blood tests, medications etc.

The cabin crew will tend to be on the aircraft early to make sure everything is in place ready to receive the passengers, likewise, the nurses and perfusionists will be in theatre early getting it ready for the patient to arrive.

One of the big decisions the captain has to make is how much fuel to take on. It costs to carry fuel, so the captain has to take a host of factors into consideration such as headwind speed, potential traffic at the destination airport and potential delay to landing. In some areas of the world, fuel is so expensive it is sometimes cheaper to carry it out with you than buy it at the destination.

In theatre, the surgeon must always have a supply of the patient's blood type available to him in case of an emergency. The surgeon will decide on how many units depending on the procedure, patient condition and the potential need for a transfusion.

A briefing of all the crew will take place in the crew room or on the plane this is the time for informing all crew members of the special needs and requirements for that particular flight.

Surgeons will have a full briefing with the theatre team on the patient and procedure just prior to commencement.

On take-off and landing, flight crews have what they call a 'sterile flight deck', up to 10,000 feet. What this means is flight commands only until they pass the 10,000ft threshold.

Although surgeons don't have such a curfew, there are times when silence is required and although this could be at any time during the procedure everyone seems to have a sixth sense when it is required.

On reaching the final destination, pilots have to do a written report on the flight and the flight crew have to check that all equipment is returned to its original position and nothing is missing.

In theatre, the surgeon will have to do a full report on the procedure which will go into the patients' notes and another copy will go into a central information database recording the surgeon's performance. The nurses have to account for every swab, stitch and instrument to avoid the possibility of things being left inside a patient. To do this they count each item, so it matches the starting numbers.

This reminded me of that great quote by the news reporter Brian Hanrahan during the Falklands War when he said, "I am not allowed to say how many planes were involved but I counted them out......and I counted them all back in."

So, we have heard from the airline pilots but what about the journey to becoming a cardiac surgeon?

One of the first people I met on my first visit to see a cardiac procedure was registrar Ms Gill Hardman. She was a trainee surgeon under the guidance of Mr Bose, the surgeon who did my procedure.

Ms Hardman is the person who gave me my first view of a beating human heart, something that will live with me for the rest of my time on the 'Circle of Life'.

I have got to know Ms Hardman over the period I have been attending theatre. She has become a great supporter and help in developing the 'Buddy Beat' concept.

In one of our many conversations, I asked her what her journey to becoming a surgeon was like.

Registrar Gill Hardman – Her story
Born in Preston to Lancastrian parents. Gill's dad failed his 11 plus and went out to work because he needed to. She is obviously very proud of her dad as she talks about what a clever man, he was but unfortunately the opportunities didn't come his way.

In a very passionate voice, she tells me he had an amazing work ethic and instilled in her if you wanted to do well you needed to work hard. That is how he lived his life and climbed up the ladder of the Xerox organisation.

Her mum, again very working-class, stacked shelves in Asda, worked as a dinner lady and a cleaner.

One of her earliest recollections of knowing what she wanted to do was to get away from Preston and where is she working now? In Blackpool, less than a handful of miles from Preston!

Ms. Hardman is an only child and the first one in her extended family to go to university. At the age of seven, she knew she wanted to be a surgeon.

She tells of a story about when she went with her dad to a BUPA hospital. A Stately Home type of place with a big Mahogany desk, leather chairs and posh cars in the car park. Her dad was to see an orthopaedic surgeon. What she saw was a very important man in a smart suit and thought this looks good. So, she decided she wanted to be an orthopaedic surgeon.

When she got home, she told her mum she had decided on her career. Her mum's response was a little less enthusiastic and said, "You have to be very clever to be a doctor. People like us don't become doctors."

One of the most inspirational elements of this story is she was never in the top sets for subjects at school. All her teachers told her she wasn't bright enough to become a doctor, even though she got great grades in her GCSE's.

At this point in her life, boys and alcohol were discovered resulting in not getting great grades in her A level exams. Although she wanted to go to university in London, her grades were not good enough and had to rely on the clearing system to be offered a place at Liverpool where she studied physiology and biomedical science. This was just part of the route to get to medical school.

This route meant at least two degrees which in this day and age with the tuition fee system would have been nigh on impossible. Fortunately, Ms Hardman's parents continued to work hard to pay for her tuition. (The financial outlay is a strong reason why so many talented working-class kids don't get the opportunity to develop their skills).

On completion of the degree, she decided to take a year out and went to Central America. She worked in a *children's cancer hospital where she learnt Spanish. During this trip, she got mugged twice at gunpoint.*

She returned to England and took up the post of HCA (health care assistant). She did this for about five years whilst she continued to study and then applied to medical school and got two offers, both in London.

Although she loved Medical School, she was never a top performer, always achieving just over the pass mark in exams. What she did do was work in a hospital several times a week as an HCA. Not only did she do the normal HCA duties of filling water jugs, changing beds she would follow doctors around and help them take blood, do ECG's and other tasks that needed doing.

She got a job mopping floors at the Royal London Hospital. She did this for three years and acquired a massive insight and access into every form of surgical speciality undertaken and their key players. They would invite her into the theatre every time there was a trauma.

At this point in our conversation, her bleep went off and she rushes to the phone to see what the requirement is. Fortunately, it was just the ward requesting a bit of information, so we return to the story.

The next disappointment was not too far away! Desperately wanting to stay in London, the system for junior foundation doctors is nationwide and based on a point scoring system. You have to put your preferred location down first and then lesser interesting locations follow. Ms. Hardman got a post in East Anglia, a part of the UK she did not know. She was so devastated to leave London that she cried for three days.

One of the jobs offered was at the world-famous Papworth Hospital, the biggest cardiothoracic hospital in the country. Here she felt there were people similar to her and struck up a friendship with another female registrar who she still keeps in touch with.

At Papworth, she decided to print off the surgeon application form, which tells you all the areas you need to fulfil to become a surgeon. This ended up on the fridge. The qualities required were highlighted and became the target for her to develop over the next couple of years.

After four years at Papworth, she applied for and got a training number, something every surgeon needs to acquire in order to be able to get a job. When applying for a job, you can only request a geographical location or hospital and Ms. Hardman got a post…in Blackpool, just a few miles from where she grew up. That was in 2014. Since then, she has worked in Alder Hay, South Manchester Hospital and then back to Blackpool which she says is starting to feel like home.

Ms. Hardman's journey to achieve her dream has not come without its challenges. She told me that in her late twenties when her friends would work during the week and then socialise at the weekend, she would either be working or studying.

Over a four-year period, she moved to a new city every six months which meant relationships were very hard to maintain. During my time visiting the cardiac centre, Ms Hardman applied for a surgeon's position in Newcastle. Apparently, there were many applicants. The panel who interviewed them had already decided on who they were going to take on, a young surgeon within their own team. That was until they met Ms Hardman who obviously impressed them to such an extent, they offered her the job. Which comes as no surprise to me!

I wanted to know more about women in powerful positions. I found a fascinating article by Hilary Clinton which made me question the differing gender make up of male and females. The quote was made when she was Secretary of State in the Obama government.

Here's what she said:

> 'At this point in my career, I have employed so many young people and one of the differences is that whenever I would say to a young woman, "I want you to do this, I want you to take on this extra responsibility, I want you to move up," invariably, they would say, "Do you think I can?" or "Do you think I have the experience?" Hilary's response was, "Well, I wouldn't be asking you if I didn't think you could and that you were ready"
>
> When I ask a young man if he wanted to move up, he would say, "How high, how fast, when do I start" There is just a hesitancy still in women's worth and work ethic that we are going to have to continue to address so more young women feel free to pursue their own ambitions and be successful.'

During my early visits, in the cardiac theatre corridor, I was told of a second young female registrar surgeon. I am told she is very quiet and timid. I have said hello on a couple of occasions but that's about it. I hear Ms. Toolan's training time in Blackpool is drawing to an end. I need to interview her and get her story so far, so we agree to meet.

Registrar Caroline Toolan – Her story
She was born in New Zealand and came to England when she was very young.

Her mum was the first one in the family to go to university, her dad also went to university but only after meeting her mum.

From an early age, Ms. Toolan found she liked all the science subjects such as biology and had a fascination for TV programmes like Casualty.

Soon, people started to realise that maybe she would be suited to medical school. So, she set about doing a number of work experience jobs including working at a vet.

Ms. Toolan found out that she enjoyed working with people and in a team.

She got the grades to get her into Medical school and spent five years in Birmingham getting trained. Her first job was in London. After a number of other jobs, she applied to do surgical training and decided cardiothoracic surgery was where she wanted to be. She had also had interests in intensive care and anaesthetics.

Ms Toolan went into surgery with her eye's wide open. She understood the stresses and strains of the training, the long hours and the duration it would take to get qualified.

I was interested in Caroline's view of being one of the few females in what could be considered as a very male-dominated environment. She said most of her training had been with white males and they had only ever given her encouragement and support. She did mention though as you climb the ladder, you do see elements that the old boys club still exists. Although not obvious, it exists through occasionally being excluded from meetings. As she put it, it's like a friendship group you're just, not part of.

Caroline is convinced that more and more women will enter this channel of surgery and that it will have universal acceptance and will be a good thing for cardiac surgery.

Although she has identified there is a differential, Caroline has the management skills to identify with and find solutions to the blockage without making it a 'gender' issue. She also identifies that the 'male domination' comes from historical culture and socialisation where the man was always the hunter-gatherer. Nowadays, she reckons that women make much better hunters.

I ask Ms. Toolan what the meaning of life is. I love asking this question to very intelligent people because they can overthink it. We have a laugh as I quote the first verse of the Lion King 'Circle of Life' and get it wrong. Ms. Toolan, the smart lady she is, was able to recite it perfectly.

The meaning of life apparently is 'a shared life'. I ask her to expand. Her response is that we are all on a journey, but it means nothing unless you can share it. Great answer!

This is one very impressive lady! A lady who has always known what she wanted to do and how to get there. So, the question of where you will be in ten years' time got the same assured and confident answer. ''In ten years, I would like to be specialising in Mitral valvular, or valvular minimal access surgery, explore robotic surgery and be able to 'fix up' the inside of the heart very reliably.''

I mentioned the potential of management and again, she has very strong views on this, saying it's all rolled into one. You can't have a well-functioning department without good leadership.

She is anything but shy and reserved as I had been told by others. She clearly knows where she is going in life and has the skills set to make it happen.

If the future of the NHS is based on young female surgeons like Gill Hardman and Caroline Toolan, then be assured, the future of our health service will be in great shape.

After much research and many conversations, I don't believe there is a defined answer to why there are so few females in cardiac surgery. There are the stereotypical answers such as motherhood etc.

I think there are three factors coming into play on this issue.

Firstly, as children, we get exposed to animals early and that's why so many want to become vets. I guess at an early age we may also visit the dentist, although the experience would surely alienate you from wanting to be one... clearly not.

Secondly, as youngsters, hopefully we never need to know anything about heart disease, so we don't have any exposure to it.

Thirdly, medical schools are now experiencing a massive rise in female students. During my many months visiting the cardiac centre, all three trainee surgeons have been female so maybe this highlights a trend that because the training is so long, some 10 to 20yrs, we are only just seeing the change in culture and the rise in female cardiac surgeons.

I believe we should be recruiting people who have the skills set to deliver in the role, male or female, it should not be about equality or a PC issue.

Here endeth the ramblings of a grumpy old man!

Reader Question

Think of the most influential women in your life.

What qualities that these women show would you like to be able to demonstrate?

Epilogue

The Journey's Conclusions

On life's journey....... to arrive as late as possible at the final destination

The idea of the book was to help me understand the cardiac journey I had been on and hopefully to inform others how a life-threatening journey can be the most inspirational one you could ever undertake. So many patients have told me their view on life is much more positive post-procedure. They now have a new lease of life and a desire to 'live it'.

As mentioned in the Prologue, I undertook this journey, not for financial gain, but by helping just one person get through a traumatic time would be the best return on investment I could ever achieve.

I had no idea or any skills on how to write a book. What I didn't want to do was write something that was boring and uninteresting. I got my inspiration from the Frank Sinatra classic and did it 'My Way.'

One thing I am proud of, is that the book has been written, quite literally, from the heart and with a passion that has inspired me and hopefully the few people that read it to realise that life is precious and very short.

On looking back at the book's journey, something that was planned to be concluded in a matter of months has now turned into a marathon and taken many, many thousands of hours. I have been up at silly o'clock to take the hour plus journey to the cardiac centre to meet patients on their arrival to have their procedure. I have seen them in surgery and witnessed every day magic conducted by some of the most brilliant magicians or artists on the planet.

I love being around highly intelligent people although the intellectual gap between us is huge. I have loved the many interviews I have done and getting behind the consultant veneer and finding the real person and their incredible motivations and ability to do what they do. I feel honoured and flattered that they have allowed me that privilege.

I have had to close the door to my home office on many occasions as I have spent many an hour sobbing my heart out when writing my experiences up. Seeing a fellow human being on the operating table motionless whilst a team of very dedicated individuals fix their heart is very humbling and extremely emotional. Surgeons cannot be emotional, it's not a characteristic that fits well with the job. But I do believe that behind the mask, they experience the spectrum of emotions we all might in these situations.

For me, understanding the journey from first-hand experience, gives me a unique relationship with the patient on the table and the family outside who are waiting to hear the news that everything went well.

As mentioned, once the book journey started, I kept meeting fascinating people with amazing stories who took me off on detours and showed me so much kindness and interest in what I was doing.

The journey kept getting extended with these many unexpected detours on the way. Hearing their amazing stories changed the focus of the book slightly to look at life and where cardiac surgery can be very inspirational within it.

I believe life isn't something that happens to us, it's what we decide life will be for us. Hours, days, weeks, months and years can be wasted thinking we still have plenty left in the tank. As Antonio Banderas said, a heart attack was the best thing to ever happen to him because he saw it as a wake-up call.

As quoted earlier in the book, Marcus Aurelius said, "We *should not fear death... what we should fear is not having lived.*"

The most powerful learning to come out of this journey is making the most of the life we have been given before it's too late. As Steve Jobs said on his death bed, "I now realise life is much more than fame and fortune."

Getting to know and understand the people and procedures available to us, should we need the help of a cardiac team, has been a once-in-a-lifetime' experience. The team at the Lancashire Cardiac Centre are world-class and I don't use term that lightly. Thirty years' experience in working with many of the top corporate teams across the globe has given me an insight into individuals, teams, communication, and performance. I have never met a team that is so passionate, committed and dedicated to the cause. The patient-centric is their core business, the focus never deviates and the desire to keep improving is a daily challenge.

Every visit to the cardiac department was a privilege. I believe this project is the first of its kind in letting a patient have an all-access pass to clinical areas and the ability to acquire intimate interviews with some of the country's top cardiac professionals. Those interviews were challenging in that this old man was suddenly in front of world-class health professionals who were expecting me to sound intelligent and in control of what I was doing.

For all those who did give me very candid, open and very honest interviews, I am eternally grateful. For those, I didn't get to interview, let's just say you have had a very lucky escape.

My 'Life's Journey began on the second of January 1950, seventy years ago. I have lived in six different decades.

Over dinner, the other night, Jerry a friend of mine of a similar age and I were discussing whether we are privileged to have lived in this era. We looked back at the sixties and agreed this was the dawn of adventure. This was the era when Britain became great again with the creation of the Beatles and the whole Mersey Beat phenomenon. The world's attention was also on Britain not only for music, as London became the global fashion centre and every blue-blooded male teenager paid homage to Mary Quant for creating the mini skirt.

The drug culture was born, and many musicians used it to create some of the most iconic songs to have ever been written. I remember going to all-night discos at the Chateau Ipney near Worcester. Thankfully, our mothers would never find out what went on at these.

The Labour government at the time, led by Harold Wilson was pretty stable and the economy was in great shape. England won the World Cup and the Americans put a man on the moon.

Jerry and I then fast-forwarded to today's youngsters and compared their lifestyle to ours. The generations are so far removed from each other. Today's youngster has all the techno-gadgets that Jerry and I have no chance of understanding. Mobile phones that can do so much more than just make a phone call. If you had talked about some of these gadgets back in the sixties, you would not have believed them to be possible.

So, today's generation has all the techno gismo's but in our dinosaur view, they also have so much more pressure on them. In the sixties, we didn't have the pressures of global warming, girl power, equality, the problems with plastic and the threats of ISIS. All these may have been around in the sixties but with the global media that exists today, all these issues are beamed into our lounges for us to worry about.

One thing I am delighted happened to me in this later generation and not in the sixties, is having cardiac disease. As mentioned, the survival rate for elective heart surgery today is around 98%. Back in the sixties, I would probably have died.

Over seventy years, I have had some amazing highs. For example, Helen and I have three amazing children who have turned out to be incredibly successful. I represented Great Britain at canoeing when I was just eighteen years old. Helen and I built a very successful corporate motivation business, working with some of the most successful brands on the planet, working in more than thirty locations around the world. I have had the honour to have worked with the England World Cup squad and had a very humbling experience to be invited by Star Wars creator George Lucas to his Skywalker Ranch in northern California to explore the potential of a global commercial project.

I have made a handful of TV documentaries, one of them, a major project involving the Calgary Stampede in Canada. Known around the world as 'The Greatest Outdoor Show in the World'

I have also met some of the most inspirational people on the planet from Apollo astronauts, George Lucas, to the man who has left a lasting impression on me, the late, great Sir Bobby Robson, England football manager. His question 'Who motivates the motivator?' to me, when we were walking around the Ipswich Town FC stadium, is a question I often ask people at the top of their game, like cardiac surgeons.

The lows in my life are probably even more spectacular, in that I lost interest in the corporate motivation business, so it failed catastrophically, and we lost our £1 million plus home and all the toys that went with it. When we reluctantly had to vacate the property, Helen and I were so sad, we got drunk for a week trying to shutout what had just happened.

As a man, I took this failure very personally. I went into a deep depression, needing professional psychiatric help. I stared at a wall for eighteen months feeling very sorry for myself. It was only when one of my daughters said to me, "What about us, daddy?" that made me realise life is not about big houses, posh cars and flaky friends who soon desert you when you no longer have a successful image. From that moment, I decided to start winning again. But winning in a different arena to the one I had been competing in previously.

As we travel on the circle of life or we rise and fall on the heartbeat of life, one thing we do not know is what is happening inside us. As the years pass by, outwardly, the wrinkles start to appear. The ageing process is there every time we look in the mirror. It's only when we start to feel unwell that it suddenly dawns on us that our inner organs are also ageing.

As we get older, the risk of getting one of the two biggest killers, heart disease or cancer, increases. Suddenly, being out of breath becomes a lot more than just being unfit. Or the lump in your breast isn't the cist you thought it was. These two killers don't discriminate as many rich and famous celebrities would testify.

My cardiac journey started back in 2012 when I first noticed something was not quite right. But my real journey started on the third of January

2017 when I had my heart surgery. This is when I realised that life is a journey with only one destination. A journey we can suddenly get to the end of and wish we had visited more locations and had far more experiences on the way.

As Steve Jobs once said, we can get so focussed on one element, in his case the desire to become rich and famous, that we miss what life's journey is really about.

Billy Connolly one of Britain's funniest comedians sees getting old as a comedy sketch as he says, "It's like someone saying I gave you all these talents when you were born and now it's time to take them back."

When we go on holiday, the destination is the exciting bit. It's where we have chosen to go. We can't wait to get there. But in life, we want to be on the journey for as long as we can before reaching the final destination.

I will never forget the privilege of the hours spent in theatre watching surgeons giving new life to very poorly people. Another day in the office for the cardiac team; a very different and life-changing one for the patient.

For Jenny, the perfusionist who said she had never had a 'thank you' card from a patient in more than twenty years of service, I hope this record continues. Not because I am a miserable old man, but because you should remain as the unsung heroes of a very dynamic team.

Although the patients may never get to know you personally, you have the incredible knowledge that you have touched each and every one of your patient's hearts and given them new life. They will always be eternally grateful for that. Surely that is the ultimate 'thank you' that you could ever wish to receive.

I refer back to the time I spent looking at the incredible homes of the rich and famous on YouTube to then walking into the living room to see the lives of Syrian's living in war-torn devastation. It just made me realise the diversity of life and went part way to answering the question, does where we are born and grow up affect who we become.

In my opinion, stress, worry, emotional and financial pressure over a long period of time can raise the chances of being diagnosed with one of the two illnesses that kill one in four of us. That said, with the dedication of the healthcare professionals I have been highly privileged to have spent time with, means the future survival rates of cardiac surgery will continue to improve.

From the dawn of humanity, we have been identifying the impossible and solving it. Think of the Wright brothers highlighted in an earlier chapter. Only birds could fly, humans couldn't. But they became famous for finding a solution to the impossible.

It was impossible to get to the top of Everest until Hillary did it in 1953. Since then, more than 4,000 individuals have achieved that definition of the impossible. Cardiac surgery is in great shape right now thanks to individuals who have achieved the impossible.

Although a cure for cancer has not yet been found, surely with the human desire to make the impossible possible, it's only a matter of time before cancer becomes a challenge overturned by the spirit of the human race.

So, as I conclude the last few paragraphs of the book, I feel as a person I have changed dramatically. Physically, I am different in that I now have a heart that works efficiently and will hopefully, keep beating for many years to come. I hope this will be the case because I now have a new respect for life, I feel in some small way, I have realised why we have been given this unique opportunity, it has given me an incredible insight into life.

I believe this journey has given me the inspiration and hopefully others to want to achieve so much more in the time we have on the 'Circle of Life.'

Life will always continue to challenge us, like today when my phone decided it wasn't going to charge. Now, as an old man, I don't need a fancy phone, but that said, I realised that even to replace the one I have, would still cost around £150. As I entered the Vodafone shop, I had accepted the need to invest in a new one. Explaining my dilemma to the assistant, they reached into a drawer and took out a tired-looking toothbrush. With a few sharp brushes over the charging point, the phone suddenly burst into life again. *'Result'* I thought, as I drove home. As soon as I entered the house, Helen told me her car had a flat tyre, an issue that cost the £150 I thought I had saved.

Material things have become much less important to me, Often, Helen and I comment on having such beautiful surroundings on our doorstep. We live in a small, fairly remote Lakeland cottage in Cumbria, where we can go for great walks with the dogs directly from our front door. It's priceless.

In an earlier chapter, Steve, our Everest marathon runner, said he would not swap his lifestyle of being a mountain guide for a multi-million-pound house and all the toys on the shores of Windermere. We all put different values on what is important in life.

Striving to do the best for your family does unfortunately, in the current world we live in, require a level of financial security, until an alternative (the impossible) can be found. Until then, Ellen Goodman's view of normal will continue to be the reality. Here's a recap.

"Normal is getting dressed in clothes that you buy for work, driving through traffic in a car that you are still paying for - in order to get to the job you need so you can pay for the clothes and the car, and the house you leave vacant all day so you can afford to live in it."

One person who has been a major mover and shaker in making my journey happen is Jordan, Mr Walker's secretary. Jordan is an incredible human being, academic and big supporter of this book. He has a degree in phenomenology (I didn't know what it meant either). I asked Jordan to put a Phenomenologists slant on life.

Here's his take on the subject.

"Rather than just thinking about things or analysing them, phenomenology is an attempt to grasp life as it is lived. In a nutshell, however, we might consider it an attempt to rouse us from stewing in our imaginations – from all the what if's and dreams about tomorrow which snatches us away from the living moment. So rather than indulging in morbid thoughts about our mortality, phenomenologists want to lead us to realise our short moment for what it is - a call to live, to be present, however, we respond to that call."

Like all of the patients I have spoken to, I didn't want to be diagnosed with a heart condition. I most definitely did not want to go through the trauma of heart surgery. But the alternative was sooner rather than later, my heart would give up on me and my life would end earlier than I had planned.

Trauma can have an amazingly positive effect. It can shake us out of that limbo we can find ourselves in, where each day is the same, undynamic and ineffective. Those days turn into weeks and the weeks turn into years, as the Pink Floyd song highlights;

And then one day you find
Ten years have got behind you
No-one told you when to run
You missed the starting gun

Suddenly, health throws you a curveball and we suddenly assess what we have done with our lives. You wish you could have all those years back so you can use them to be more effective or as the song says, *'see more and do more.'*

Every year has 365 days, excluding leap years. Yet we have very little recall on what we were doing on any one of those days. It's only the days that something significant happened that we remember. One of my missions going forward is to remember more of the 365 days for achieving something remarkable or at least memorable.

Helen and I own a reasonably successful Selfie Mirror/Photobooth hire business where we go to weddings and celebrations and take silly photos of people dressed up in the props we supply.

Last weekend, I did an event for a thirteenth birthday party, attended by thirty teenagers. They dressed up in the props we provided, looked in the mirror and took selfies. When I looked in the mirror, I saw the massive generation gap.

At thirteen, you have the security of your family and home; life is just one big adventure. At one point, I got talking to the birthday girl's dad and said, 'oh to be thirteen again,' to which he replied 'yep, they have no idea of what life is going to throw at them in the future. For now, life is just continuous fun.' Life-threatening illness, financial and relationship pressures are not on their radar. I wonder where life's journey will take them.

One of my motivations to write this book was because I went through a very negative period after my procedure. When I looked for support and information, I felt there was little to help me understand what I was feeling. I wanted to know if other patients felt what I was feeling and how did they handle it. Unfortunately, I could not find answers to my many questions, hence the need to write this book in an attempt to answer some of those questions and hopefully, help others with a similar need.

An area I feel is a major challenge for the NHS is identifying the emotional journey patients undertake with major surgery or illness. The physical, medication and physiotherapy paths are seen as the core areas for recovery with the enormous investment made into improving them. But what about the emotional journey. In my opinion as a patient, this is an area so critical to recovery and wellbeing yet is not recognised as the third major strand in patient care and rehabilitation., This is still an area unavailable to patients.

'Buddy Beat' is my idea of creating a professionally trained team of post-operative 'buddies' who can be made available to buddy new patients who are about to take on the journey. The aim is to be there when the patient needs them and to help them on the emotional rollercoaster.

At present, we are trying to form a team of highly qualified health professionals and academics with the aim of developing a three-year funded project to evaluate the emotional and physical benefits to the patients of having a professional 'Buddy Beat' support group.

So, after more than two years on this amazing journey, what conclusions have I come to.

We've already discovered if you asked all eight billion people who inhabit the planet to interpret life, you would get eight billion different interpretations. But is there a life model that we would all be happy with. One we could be happy and content to live within. I doubt it because what makes the human race so fascinating is, we are all uniquely wired. Our fantastic ability and inquisitiveness to resolve the impossible is also the same drive that creates tension, hatred and discord. As one Apollo astronaut said, looking down at the beauty of our blue planet, 'why can't we all live in harmony with each other.'

How can we inject more laughter and fun into our lives? After all, they are a physiological requirement for all of mankind.

As the lord said to Adam, I have given you something much more powerful than 'fight or flight,' I have given you a sense of humour. Patch Adams has believed this and practised it all his life. Science and the academic world agree and endorse the powerful health benefits of humour.

I went to see Ben Fogle the TV presenter and adventurer who was doing a show in Blackpool. Ben has a fascinating philosophy on life: he says you have to 'complete not compete'. A fascinating approach to life and not one many Olympic athletes would agree to but for the many millions of us who aren't Olympic athletes, then I guess he is saying whatever you start in life, make sure you finish it. In other words, keep going until its finished.

Coming full circle, life-threatening illness can give you the same inspirational life-changing view on life as a lottery win can. We suddenly realise life is not forever and we need to maximise the time we have left. It has certainly done that for me and many of the patients I have been privileged to meet on this most amazing journey.

Maybe the best way of concluding the journey is with something I have very strong feelings on, it is;

We enter this world with nothing.........
and we leave it with nothing
But the bit in-between is our very own
unique personal journey.
Put your heart and soul into life...... while
you still have it.